Idiopathic Granulomatous Mastitis

Hande Koksal • Naim Kadoglou

Editors

Idiopathic Granulomatous Mastitis

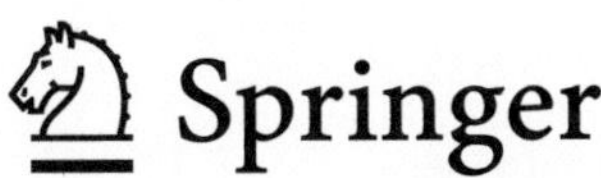 Springer

Editors
Hande Koksal
Department of General Surgery
Selcuk University, Faculty of Medicine
Konya, Türkiye

Naim Kadoglou
Imperial Collage, Breast Unit, London
North West University Healthcare NHS
Trust, Northwick Park Hospital, Harrow
London, UK

ISBN 978-3-031-30393-7   ISBN 978-3-031-30391-3   (eBook)
https://doi.org/10.1007/978-3-031-30391-3

This Springer imprint is published by the registered company Springer Nature Switzerland AG
The registered company address is: Gewerbestrasse 11, 6330 Cham, Switzerland

Foreword

Idiopathic Granulomatous Mastitis (IGM) is a difficult condition both for patients and their physicians. Usually in medicine a doctor makes a diagnosis and having prescribed treatment, the condition improves. This is not the situation in IGM. First making the diagnosis of IGM is not always easy. Malignancy is often the initial diagnosis, and the full range of pathological changes described in IGM is not always all present in all patients. The clinical presentation of IGM also overlaps with the clinical features of tuberculosis so excluding TB by sending biopsies for culture is important in such patients before making the diagnosis of IGM. Second, once a diagnosis is made there is no established treatment. Third, there is no established aetiology. Fourth, the clinical course of IGM is variable.

With so much unknown and so much controversy in the literature about IGM, this book is exactly what clinicians and patients have needed for some time. The authors discuss all the information available on IGM covering the clinical features, aetiology, and treatment. It is comprehensive, well balanced and it has a comprehensive list of references at the end of each chapter.

I enjoyed reading this book and liked the way it is laid out into small easy digestible chapters dealing with all the major issues in relation to IGM. The chapter on the role of infection in this condition was a particular favourite of mine. The section on aetiology includes new data on the role of different subsets of inflammatory cells and discusses whether IGM has an underlying autoimmune component.

I have treated many women with this condition. I used to use steroids to treat IGM but now rarely use these. The authors note that most cases resolve with a conservative approach making sure any abscesses are appropriately treated by aspiration or by small incision drainage. I have seen more patients who have had problems after surgery than I have seen helped by surgery. The section on treatment in this book is comprehensive and makes the very important point that there is no one best treatment for all patients with this condition.

It is a great privilege and pleasure to recommend this book to all involved in managing this very difficult condition. The authors have done a fantastic job of summarizing all that is known and have made it easy to read and digest. Prepare to be much more knowledgeable about IGM at the end of this book than you are now.

Mike.Dixon@ed.ac.uk   Mike J. Dixon
Breakthrough Breast Cancer Research Unit
University of Edinburgh, Western General Hospital
Edinburgh, UK

Acknowledgement

The authors would like to thank Miss Edagül Uluçay, B.Sc. for taking the time to proofread and edit the manuscript. Edagül is a 5th year medical student studying at Imperial College School of Medicine (ICSM) London. She is currently undertaking a bioengineering PhD looking at redefining photodynamic therapy of cancers using bioharmonophores, a new class of optical imaging nanoprobe.

Contents

Contributors

Shyamala Fernandez, MD Department of Pathology, Ealing Hospital, London North West University Healthcare NHS Trust, London, UK

Natalie G. Johnson, MBBS, FRCS (Eng), PhD The Royal Marsden Hospital, London, UK

Naim Kadoglou, MD, FRCS Imperial College, Breast Unit, London North West University Healthcare NHS Trust, Northwick Park Hospital, Harrow, London, UK

Hande Koksal, MD, FEBS, FACS Department of General Surgery, Selcuk University, Faculty of Medicine, Konya, Türkiye

Mia Morgan, MD Department of Radiology, London North West University Healthcare NHS Trust, Northwick Park Hospital, London, UK

Leyla Ozer, MD, PhD, EBMG Department of Medical Genetics, Faculty of Medicine, Yuksek Ihtisas University, Ankara, Türkiye

Microgen Genetic Diagnostic Centers, Ankara, Türkiye

Nevin Sekmenli, MD Department of Radiology, Saglik Bilimleri University, Hamidiye Faculty of Medicine, Ministry of Health Konya City Hospital, Konya, Türkiye

William Teh, MD Department of Radiology, London North West University Healthcare NHS Trust, Northwick Park Hospital, London, UK

Esra Yilmaz, MD Department of Pathology, Saglik Bilimleri University, Hamidiye Faculty of Medicine, Ministry of Health, Konya City Hospital, Konya, Türkiye

Overview on Idiopathic Granulomatous Mastitis

Hande Koksal (iD)

1 Introduction

Milward and Gough [1] described granulomatous lesions in the breast that were confused with breast carcinoma in 1970. The entity "idiopathic granulomatous mastitis" (IGM) was first reported by Kessler and Wolloch [2] in five cases. These patients were defined as cases with suspected breast cancer, but characterized by granulomas and abscesses on pathological examination. Later in 1977, Cohen [3] detailed this clinical entity.

Many factors such as α1-antitrypsin deficiency, oral contraceptive drug use, smoking, pregnancy, childbirth and breastfeeding, hyperprolactinemia, ethnic origin, and autoimmunity have been blamed in the etiopathogenesis of IGM until today. However, the etiopathogenesis has not been explained exactly yet. Recently, some associations and findings in IGM, such as coexistence with erythema nodosum and arthritis, which are more common in rheumatological diseases such as Sjögren's syndrome, and the increase in the use of steroids in treatment, suggest autoimmunity and immune dysregulation more likely in the etiopathogenesis [4–11].

Idiopathic granulomatous mastitis is a mysterious disease that continues to attract many researchers' attention, with many unknowns. Unfortunately, the pathogenesis and an ideal treatment approach of IGM, a disease known for nearly half a century, are still unknown. Many unknowns about the etiology of the disease also persist. For example, these questions should be answered: (i) Why is IGM more

H. Koksal (✉)
Department of General Surgery, Selcuk University, Faculty of Medicine, Konya, Türkiye

H. Koksal, N. Kadoglou (eds.), *Idiopathic Granulomatous Mastitis*,
https://doi.org/10.1007/978-3-031-30391-3_1

1

frequently observed in countries such as Turkey, China, South Korea, and Saudi Arabia? (ii) Why is it more common in premenopausal women? As emphasized above, although it has been known for half a century as a clinical entity, it still remains as a mystery.

2 Definition

There are various causes of granulomatous inflammation in the breast. The conditions that cause granulomas are shown in Table 1 [5, 12–14].

Generally, idiopathic granulomatous mastitis, a rare disease, may be confused with breast carcinomas. Patients with IGM present with a mass accompanied by inflammation manifestations such as erythema and pain. In order to diagnose IGM, histologically, there should be a non-caseous granulomatous inflammation. In addition, other causes of granulomatous inflammation should be ruled out including infectious diseases such as tuberculosis, fungi, parasites, or a systemic granulomatous disease, for example, sarcoidosis and Wegener's granulomatosis [5, 10, 12–14]. Briefly, IGM is a diagnosis of exclusion when other causes of granulomatous mastitis cannot be detected after demonstrating non-caseous granulomas histopathologically. The pathological features of IGM are discussed in detail in the "pathology and differential diagnosis" section.

Table 1 Causes of granulomatous inflammation in the breast

Causes
Infectious
Mycobacterium tuberculosis
Blastomycosis
Cryptococcosis
Histoplasmosis
Actinomycosis
Filarial infection
Corynebacterium
Autoimmune
Wegener granulomatosis
Giant cell arteritis
Foreign body reaction
Duct ectasis
Plasma cell mastitis
Subareolar granuloma
Periductal mastitis
Diabetes mellitus
Sarcoidosis
Fat necrosis
Idiopathic

3 Historical Perspective

Granulomatous mastitis was first defined by Milward and Gough [1]. In 1967, the authors performed a biopsy on a patient with a clinical suspicion of breast cancer. They froze this section; however, they could not find any evidence of carcinoma in the patient.

Pathologically, they found granulomatous inflammation in the patient. The authors retrospectively reviewed 691 patients who underwent local or radical mastectomy with a clinical diagnosis of breast cancer between 1960 and 1967 at United Oxford Hospitals. During this period, no evidence of breast carcinoma was detected in eight patients who were operated with a clinical diagnosis of breast carcinoma. The authors found a condition unlike the known noninfective inflammatory breast diseases including fat necrosis and periductal mastitis in four patients. There was a condition in the breast that was accompanied by granulomatous inflammation.

In 1972, Kessler and Wolloch [2] described five patients who were clinically similar to breast carcinoma, but had no evidence of breast carcinoma on pathological examination, similar to Milward and Gough [1]. Multiple granulomas and abscesses were observed in these patients. All patients were women in childbearing age, and they had given birth. The age of the patients was found to be between 27 and 40 years.

In two patients, a preoperative punch biopsy had been performed and they were diagnosed with carcinoma and received preoperative radiotherapy. However, as a result of the definitive surgery of these two patients, no finding of carcinoma had been found. "Lipid crystals" were investigated to rule out fat necrosis. In addition, Ziehl-Neelsen stain for acid-fast bacilli, Gram staining for bacteria, and periodic acid-Schiff reaction for fungi were used. No positivity was found in any of the patients. In conclusion, Kessler and Wolloch [2] used the term "idiopathic granulomatous mastitis" for the first time.

Cohen [3] reviewed 67 patients diagnosed with granulomatous tuberculosis, or fungal mastitis, and revealed five patients with granulomatous mastitis as described by Kessler and Wolloch [2]. The patients with granulomatous mastitis that fit the definition of Kessler and Wolloch accounted for 7.5% of all granulomatous mastitis patients. Cohen's patients were young women of childbearing age, as were the patients of Kessler and Wolloch [2]. The patients' age ranged between 17 and 34 years old. Cohen [3] described the pathological characteristics of patients with idiopathic granulomatous mastitis.

References

1. Milward TM, Gough MH. Granulomatous lesions in the breast presenting as carcinoma. Surg Gynecol Obstet. 1970;130:478–82.
2. Kessler E, Wolloch Y. Granulomatous mastitis: a lesion clinically simulating carcinoma. Am J Clin Pathol. 1972;58:642–6. https://doi.org/10.1093/ajcp/58.6.642.

3. Cohen C. Granulomatous mastitis. A review of 5 cases. S Afr Med J. 1977;52:14–6.
4. Akın M, Karabacak H, Esendağlı G, Yavuz A, Gültekin S, Dikmen K, et al. Coexistence of idiopathic granulomatous mastitis and erythemanodosum: successful treatment with corticosteroids. Turk J Med Sci. 2017;47:1590–2. https://doi.org/10.3906/sag-1611-100.
5. Altintoprak F, Kivilcim T, Ozkan OV. Aetiology of idiopathic granulomatous mastitis. World J Clin Cases. 2014;2:852–8. https://doi.org/10.12998/wjcc.v2.i12.852.
6. Benson JR, Dumitru D. Idiopathic granulomatous mastitis: presentation, investigation and management. Future Oncol. 2016;12:1381–94. https://doi.org/10.2217/fon-2015-0038.
7. Sheybani F, Naderi HR, Gharib M, Sarvghad M, Mirfeizi Z. Idiopathic granulomatous mastitis: long-discussed but yet-to-be-known. Autoimmunity. 2016;49:236–9. https://doi.org/1 0.3109/08916934.2016.1138221.
8. Vural S, Ertop P, Ceyhan K, Şanli H. An unusual cause of oligoarthritis and erythema nodosum: idiopathic granulomatous mastitis. Arch Rheumatol. 2017;32:71–5. https://doi.org/10.5606/ ArchRheumatol.2017.5952.
9. Yazigi G, Trieu BH, Landis M, Parikh JG, Mangal M. Granulomatous mastitis: a rare case with Sjogren's syndrome and complications. Cureus. 2019;11:e5359. https://doi.org/10.7759/ cureus.5359.
10. Yin Y, Liu X, Meng Q, Han X, Zhang H, Lv Y. Idiopathic granulomatous mastitis: etiology, clinical manifestation, diagnosis and treatment. J Investig Surg. 2022;35(3):709–20. https:// doi.org/10.1080/08941939.2021.1894516.
11. Zabetian S, Friedman BJ, McHargue C. A case of idiopathic granulomatous mastitis associated with erythema nodosum, arthritis, and reactive cough. JAAD Case Rep. 2016;2:125–7. https://doi.org/10.1016/j.jdcr.2016.01.011.
12. Bakaris S, Yuksel M, Ciragil P, Guven MA, Ezberci F, Bulbuloglu E. Granulomatous mastitis including breast tuberculosis and idiopathic lobular granulomatous mastitis. Can J Surg. 2006;49:427–30.
13. Hoda SA. Inflammatory and reactive tumors. In: Hoda SA, Koerner FC, Brogi E, Rosen PP, editors. Rosens's breast pathology. 4th ed. Philadelphia: Wolters Kluwer; 2015a. p. 37–77.
14. Hoda SA. Inflammatory and reactive tumors. In: Hoda SA, Koerner FC, Brogi E, Rosen PP, editors. Rosens's breast pathology. 4th ed. Philadelphia: Wolters Kluwer; 2015b. p. 79–94.

Epidemiology

Hande Koksal

1 Gender

Although idiopathic granulomatous mastitis is mostly a disease which occurs in women, it can rarely be diagnosed in men (1.4%). Except for 13 male patients emphasized by Yaghan et al. [1] after their search in PubMed databases, almost all of the patients with IGM described in literature are women [1–7].

2 Age

Idiopathic granulomatous mastitis can be seen at almost any age (Fig. 1). It is most common in premenopausal women who are childbearing. However, the male patients with IGM reported are mostly over 40 years old [1].

While IGM is usually common in women in the fourth decade (age between 30 and 40 years), it is generally seen in men older than 40 years old (Fig. 2). The probable reason for this can be attributed to the increase in estrogen in men in this age period. However, in order to conclude this with more certainty, further research of IGM in male patients is required.

H. Koksal (✉)
Department of General Surgery, Selcuk University, Faculty of Medicine, Konya, Türkiye

H. Koksal, N. Kadoglou (eds.), *Idiopathic Granulomatous Mastitis*,
https://doi.org/10.1007/978-3-031-30391-3_2

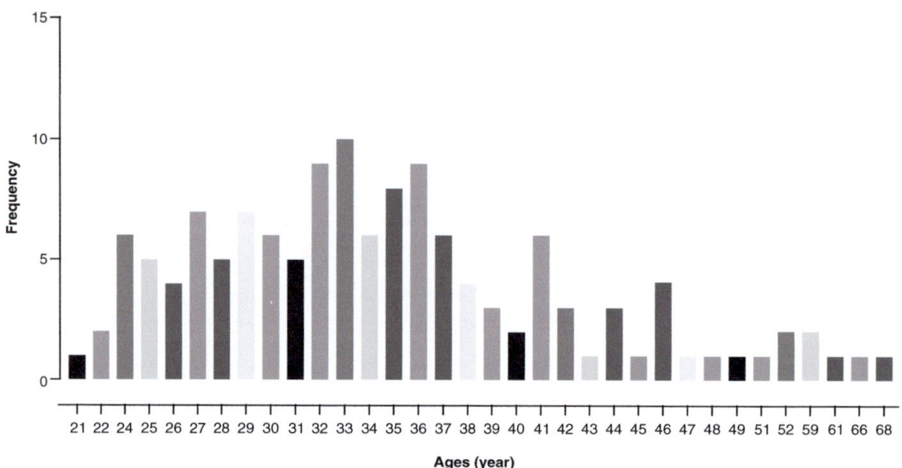

Fig. 1 The age distribution of our IGM patients

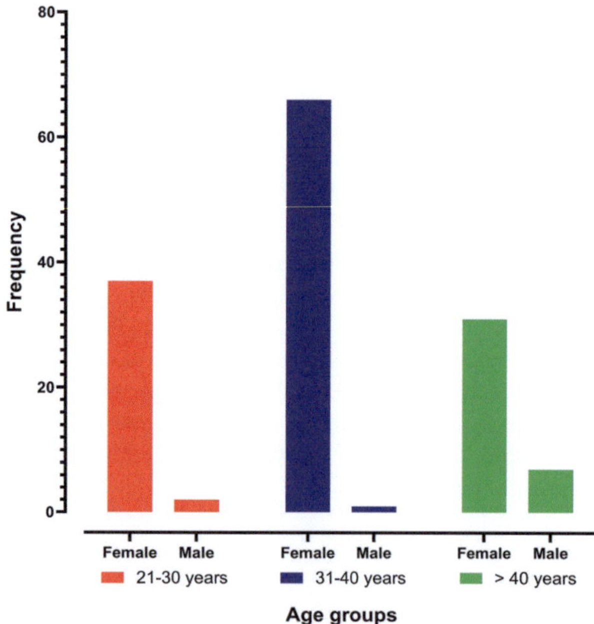

Fig. 2 Age distribution by gender

3 History of Parity and Breastfeeding

Considering the age at which idiopathic granulomatous mastitis is prevalent, it is noted that more than 90% of the patients are in the premenopausal period and a great majority of these patients are of a reproductive age (Fig. 3). When the parity

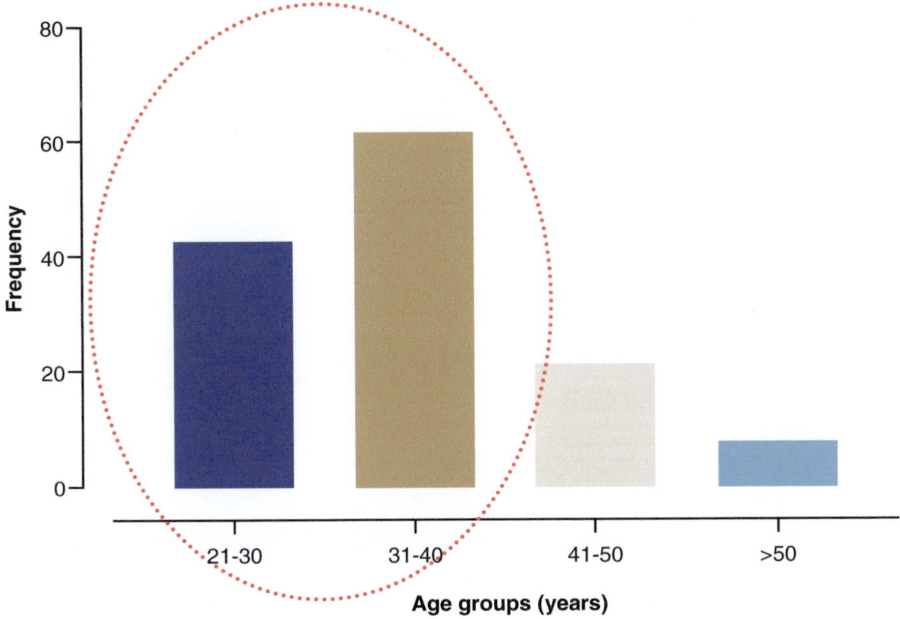

Fig. 3 Age distribution of our IGM patients

of IGM patients is examined, it is reported that 90% of the patients have a history of at least one pregnancy and this is similar in the history of breastfeeding [5, 8–10].

When the time between the onset of IGM symptoms and the last birth is evaluated, it is seen that the disease occurs after the second year of the last birth [5, 9]. However, an important point to remember is that IGM can occur at a very young age or at an advanced age, which is not related with the fertile period [5, 11]. In addition, although few, it should be noted that there are also male patients [1].

4   Ethnicity

Although idiopathic granulomatous mastitis may be seen all over the world, it is more frequent in countries such as Turkey, United States of America, China, India, Iran, and Saudi Arabia [12]. Figure 4 shows the distribution of idiopathic granulomatous mastitis-related publications by country (note: only publications in the form of research articles or case reports are included) from the PubMed database which has been schematized since 1971. The distribution of publications on IGM from countries may indirectly reflect the distribution of IGM patients.

The answer to "Why is IGM more common in these countries?" is very important in understanding the pathogenesis of idiopathic granulomatous mastitis. Another question that needs to be answered is, "is there a genetic predisposition?" In our previous study [13], we investigated the distribution of patients with human leukocyte antigens (HLA) class I and II in Turkish IGM patients, in order to answer "Why is IGM more

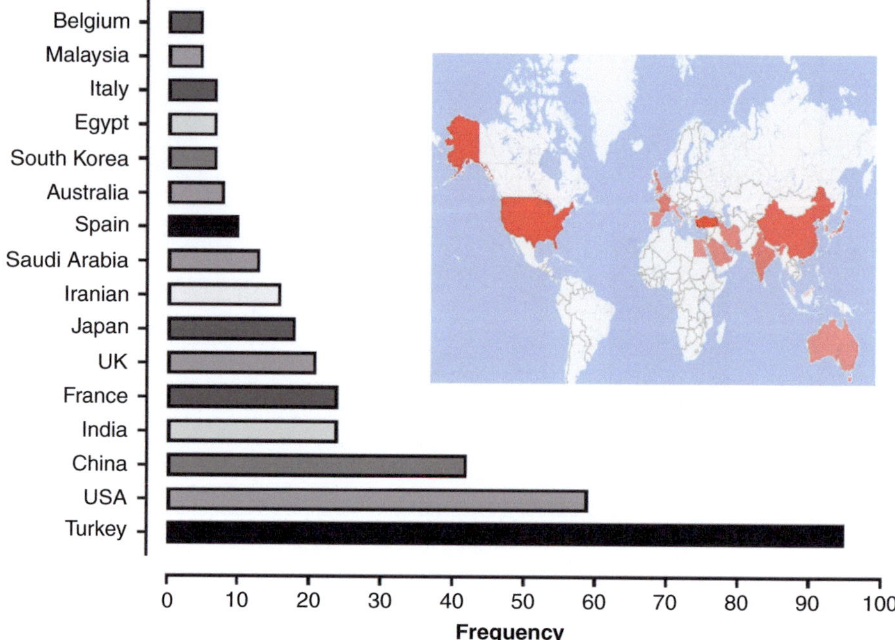

Fig. 4 The distribution of idiopathic granulomatous mastitis-related publications by country which has been schematized since 1971 (note: only publications in the form of research articles or case reports are included)

frequent in Turkey?" and "Is ethnicity an important factor in the pathogenesis?" In Turkish IGM patients, HLA-A*10, HLA-A*2403, HLA-B*18, and HLA-DR*17 antigens were higher than the control group, while HLA-A*29, HLA-B*14, and HLA-DR*1 were lower. The importance of this study will be further increased by investigating the distribution of HLA in other countries where IGM is common.

5 Place of Residence of the Patients

When the relationship between the patients' place of residence and IGM is examined, most IGM patients live in the city centers (88–95%) [5, 14].

6 Education

Uysal et al. [14] showed that 256 (42%) of 720 patients were primary school graduates and 218 (36%) were high school graduates. In this study, the rate of university graduates is low (12%). Similarly, in our study [5], the educational status of a

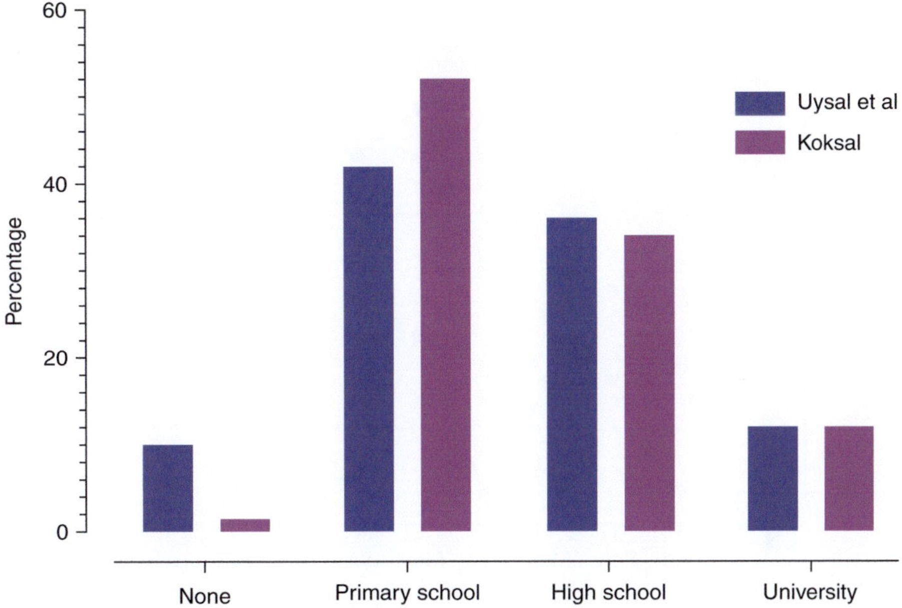

Fig. 5 The educational status of patients with idiopathic granulomatous mastitis

significant portion of the patients was primary school or high school graduates (Fig. 5).

7 Seasonal Fluctuation

A very interesting finding found in both our [5, 15] studies, published on similar dates, is the seasonal fluctuation (Fig. 6).

It is known that there are seasonal fluctuations occur in some diseases [16], such as infections (especially viral); immune-based diseases (immune dysregulation or autoimmune disease) like Kawasaki disease, vasculitis, type I diabetes mellitus in children, and idiopathic (immune) thrombocytopenia; and some malignant diseases such as Hodgkin lymphoma and skin cancers [17–24]. In both children and adults, immune thrombocytopenic purpura is more common in the spring months and during the first days of summer, which can be explained as an autoimmune disease triggered by viral infections, which are common especially in these seasonal transition periods [18, 19, 21]. It has been emphasized that there may also be seasonal fluctuations in IGM [5, 15]. The increase in the number of IGM patients in the spring months and the first days of summer (similarly to immune thrombocytopenic purpura) raises the question of whether it may also be an autoimmune disease triggered by a previous viral infection or not [5].

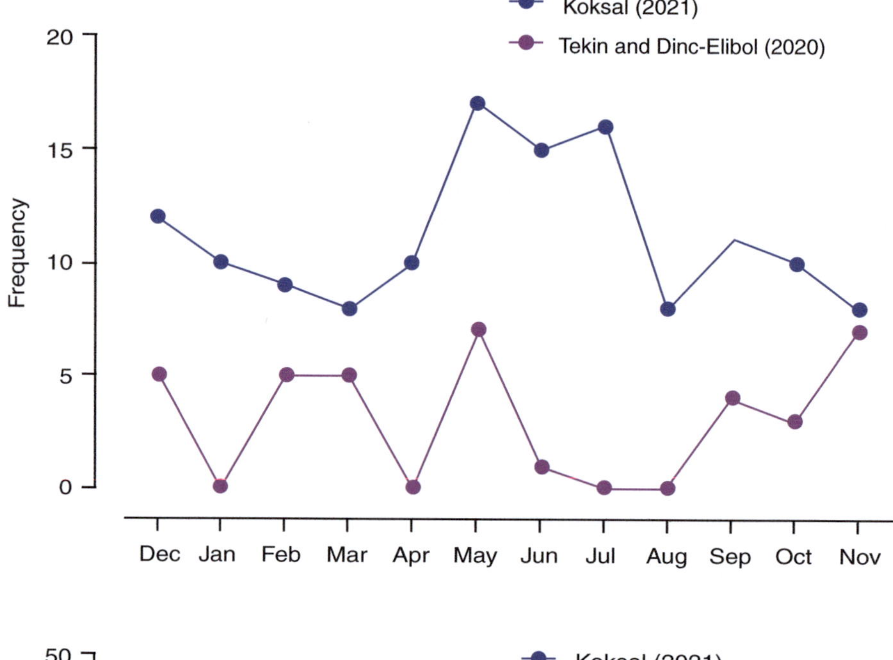

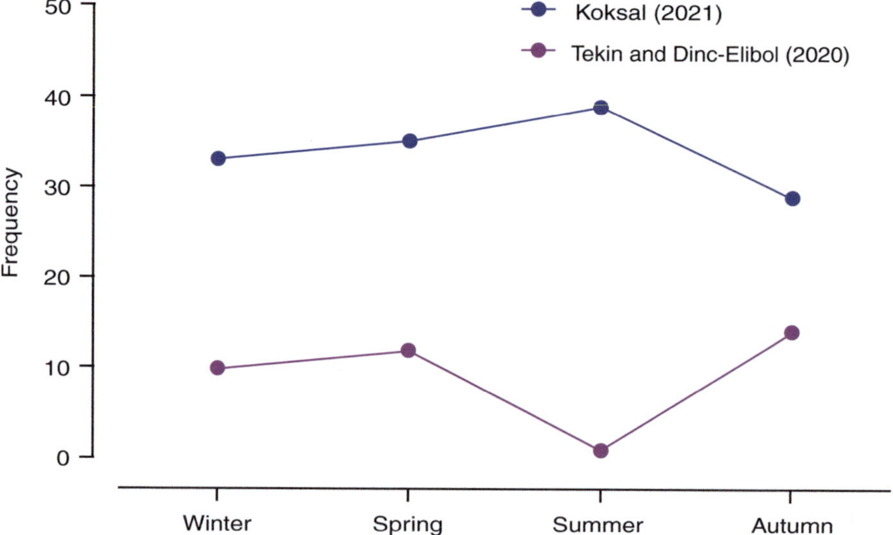

Fig. 6 The seasonal fluctuation of idiopathic granulomatous mastitis

References

1. Yaghan RJ, Ayoub NM, Shenawi HM, Yaghan LR. Idiopathic granulomatous mastitis in the male population: a clinical analysis of 13 reported cases. Breast J. 2020;26:1481–2. https://doi.org/10.1111/tbj.13778.
2. Al Manasra AR, Al-Hurani MF. Granulomatous mastitis: a rare cause of male breast lump. Case Rep Oncol. 2016;9:516–9. https://doi.org/10.1159/000448990.
3. Dinç Elibol F, Elibol C, Tekin L, Dönmez C. A very rare cause of male breast lump: idiopathic granulomatous mastitis. Breast J. 2020;26:778–9. https://doi.org/10.1111/tbj.13571.
4. Kiyak G, Dumlu EG, Kilinc I, Tokaç M, Akbaba S, Gurer A, et al. Management of idiopathic granulomatous mastitis: dilemmas in diagnosis and treatment. BMC Surg. 2014;14:66. https://doi.org/10.1186/1471-2482-14-66.
5. Koksal H. What are the new findings with regard to the mysterious disease idiopathic granulomatous mastitis? Surg Today. 2021;51:1158–68. https://doi.org/10.1007/s00595-020-02204-2.
6. Prasad S, Jaiprakash P, Dave A, Pai D. Idiopathic granulomatous mastitis: an institutional experience. Turk J Surg. 2017;33:100–3. https://doi.org/10.5152/turkjsurg.2017.3439.
7. Reddy KM, Meyer CE, Nakdjevani A, Shrotria S. Idiopathic granulomatous mastitis in the male breast. Breast J. 2005;11:73. https://doi.org/10.1111/j.1075-122X.2005.21404.x.
8. Azizi A, Prasath V, Canner J, Gharib M, Sadat Fattahi A, et al. Idiopathic granulomatous mastitis: management and predictors of recurrence in 474 patients. Breast J. 2020;26:1358–62. https://doi.org/10.1111/tbj.13822.
9. Cetinkaya G, Kozan R, Emral AC, Tezel E. Granulomatous mastitis, watch and wait is a good option. Ir J Med Sci. 2021;190:1117–22. https://doi.org/10.1007/s11845-020-02406-0.
10. Shojaee L, Rahmani N, Moradi S, Motamedi A, Godazandeh G. Idiopathic granulomatous mastitis: challenges of treatment in iranian women. BMC Surg. 2021;21:206. https://doi.org/10.1186/s12893-021-01210-6.
11. Bani-Hani KE, Yaghan RJ, Matalka II, Shatnawi NJ. Idiopathic granulomatous mastitis: time to avoid unnecessary mastectomies. Breast J. 2004;10:318–22. https://doi.org/10.1111/tbj.13822.
12. Altintoprak F, Kivilcim T, Ozkan OV. Aetiology of idiopathic granulomatous mastitis. World J Clin Cases. 2014;2:852–8. https://doi.org/10.12998/wjcc.v2.i12.852.
13. Koksal H. Human leukocyte antigens class I and II in patients with idiopathic granulomatous mastitis. Am J Surg. 2019;218:605–8. https://doi.org/10.1016/j.amjsurg.2019.01.038.
14. Uysal E, Soran A, Sezgin E, Granulomatous Mastitis Study Group. Factors related to recurrence of idiopathic granulomatous mastitis: what do we learn from a multicentre study? ANZ J Surg. 2018;88:635–9. https://doi.org/10.1111/ans.14115.
15. Tekin L, Dinç Elibol F. Is there any relationship between granulomatous mastitis and seasons? an analysis of seasonal frequency, clinical, and radiologic findings. Eur J Breast Health. 2020;16(4):235–43. https://doi.org/10.5152/ejbh.2020.5897. eCollection 2020 Oct. PMID: 33062962
16. Douglas AS, Allan TM, Rawles JM. Composition of seasonality of disease. Scott Med J. 1991;36:76–82. https://doi.org/10.1177/003693309103600304.
17. Burns JC, Herzog L, Fabri O, Tremoulet AH, Rodó X, Uehara R, et al. Seasonality of Kawasaki disease: a global perspective. PLoS One. 2013;8:e74529. https://doi.org/10.1371/journal.pone.0074529.
18. Cohn J. Thrombocytopenia in childhood: an evaluation of 433 patients. Scand J Haematol. 1976;16:226–40. https://doi.org/10.1111/j.1600-0609.1976.tb01142.x.
19. Kühne T, Imbach P, Bolton-Maggs PH, Berchtold W, Blanchette V, Buchanan GR, Intercontinental Childhood ITP Study Group. Newly diagnosed idiopathic thrombocytopenic purpura in childhood: an observational study. Lancet. 2001;358(9299):2122–5. https://doi.org/10.1016/S0140-6736(01)07219-1.

20. Morikawa S, Kohdera U, Hosaka T, Ishii K, Akagawa S, Hiroi S, et al. Seasonal variations of respiratory viruses and etiology of human rhinovirus infection in children. J Clin Virol. 2015;73:14–9. https://doi.org/10.1016/j.jcv.2015.10.001.
21. Moulis G, Guénin S, Limal N, Michel M, Bierling P, Godeau B, et al. Seasonal variations of incident primary immune thrombocytopenia in adults: an ecological study. Eur J Intern Med. 2017;37:e26–8. https://doi.org/10.1016/j.ejim.2016.09.025.
22. Newell GR, Lynch HK, Gibeau JM, Spitz MR. Seasonal diagnosis of Hodgkin's disease among young adults. J Natl Cancer Inst. 1985;74:53–6.
23. Roche EF, McKenna AM, Ryder KJ, Brennan AA, O'Regan M, Hoey HM. Is the incidence of type 1 diabetes in children and adolescents stabilising? The first 6 years of a National Register. Eur J Pediatr. 2016;175:1913–9. https://doi.org/10.1007/s00431-016-2787-6.
24. Tidman M, Olander R, Svalander C, Danielsson D. Patients hospitalized because of small vessel vasculitides with renal involvement in the period 1975-95: organ involvement, anti-neutrophil cytoplasmic antibodies patterns, seasonal attack rates and fluctuation of annual frequencies. J Intern Med. 1998;244:133–41. https://doi.org/10.1046/j.1365-2796.1998.00324.x.

Etiology and Pathogenesis

Hande Koksal and Naim Kadoglou

Since the first definition of IGM in 1971 by Kessler and Wolloch, this entity's etiology and pathogenesis have not been exactly explained yet.

Various reasons such as α1-antitrypsin deficiency; oral contraceptives; gestation, birth, and breastfeeding; hyperprolactinemia; smoking; microbial agents; ethnicity; and autoimmunity have been suggested, but have not yet been fully proved up to now [1, 2].

1 α1-Antitrypsin Deficiency

In a 37-year-old female patient diagnosed with IGM, alpha-1 antitrypsin deficiency was found on investigation. This, the first concurrent alpha-1 antitrypsin deficiency and IGM were reported [3]. However, no other publication other than this case report has been found in English literature. This association is most likely due to a coincidence.

H. Koksal (✉)
Department of General Surgery, Selcuk University, Faculty of Medicine, Konya, Türkiye

N. Kadoglou
Imperial College, Breast Unit, London North West University Healthcare NHS Trust, Northwick Park Hospital, Harrow, London, UK

© The Author(s), under exclusive license to Springer Nature Switzerland AG 2023
H. Koksal, N. Kadoglou (eds.), *Idiopathic Granulomatous Mastitis*,
https://doi.org/10.1007/978-3-031-30391-3_3

2 Oral Contraceptives

It has been suggested that oral contraceptives may play a role in the pathogenesis of IGM and this has been thought to occur as a consequence of increasing breast secretion. However, the frequency of oral contraceptive use in patients with IGM is variable (0–40%). Although it does not seem to have a direct effect, it may have a possible contribution to the pathogenesis of IGM through hormonal changes [4–9]).

3 Hyperprolactinemia

In the etiology and pathogenesis of IGM, drug-induced hyperprolactinemia and prolactinomas have been another interesting topics [10–15]. In an article from China (only the "abstract" can be obtained), high serum prolactin level was determined in 39.7% of 300 patients with granulomatous lobular mastitis [16].

Li and McGregor [14] reported a case of IGM associated with hyperprolactinemia. Their patient did not respond to antibiotic treatment; however, they did respond to bromocriptine that is used for hyperprolactinemia. Destek et al. [12] reported that their patient with IGM who did not respond to antibiotic (10 days) and steroid treatment (2 months) and then a pituitary prolactinoma was diagnosed. Cabergoline, a prolactin inhibitor, was administered for hyperprolactinemia. It was observed that IGM resolved in the fourth month of cabergoline treatment. In another case report, an IGM patient associated with risperidone-induced hyperprolactinemia is presented. The patient's risperidone treatment was changed to quetiapine and the patient's lesions resolved with steroid treatment [13].

The following questions, "Does hyperprolactinemia really play a role in IGM etiology and pathogenesis?" or "Is this union a coincidence?," should also be answered. In patients with hyperprolactinemia, most common manifestations are menstrual disturbances, weight gain, galactorrhea, headache, visual field defects, and infertility [17]. In our previous study [8], there was no symptom or sign suggestive of hyperprolactinemia. Additionally, we found that the time since the last birth ranged from 1 month to 37 years (median, 4 years) in IGM patients. When the time of IGM patients' last birth were grouped, IGM was observed after 24 months at most.

There is no such information mentioned about the number of breastfeeding patients with high prolactin levels in the article by Chen et al. [16]. Especially if the number of breastfeeding women is high, this may explain the number of women with high prolactin levels. However, all these findings are not sufficient to exactly explain the role of hyperprolactinemia in the etiology and pathogenesis of IGM.

4   Gestation, Birth, and Breastfeeding

Although IGM can be seen in both men and women at any age, it is usually seen in women who are premenopausal, are parous, and have a breastfeeding history (Fig. 1) [8, 18]. As seen in Fig. 1, the majority of IGM patients are in the reproductive age range.

Idiopathic granulomatous mastitis can be seen in women who have never been pregnant or have not given birth [10, 19, 20]. In our series, the percentage of nulliparous women was 4.5% [8].

The question "Is pregnancy an etiological factor of IGM?" does not have an exact answer. The percentage of pregnant patients with IGM at diagnosis was 4.5% [8]. However, there may be a triggering factor [21]. Sener Bahce and Aktas [22] reviewed 35 IGM patients. They reported that four of six patients with erythema nodosum and arthritis were pregnant at the time of IGM diagnosis.

In addition, the percentage of pregnant and breastfeeding patients at IGM diagnosis were 4.5% and 3.7%, respectively [8]. While these rates may give a doubtful impression about the role of pregnancy in the etiopathogenesis of IGM, it shows that extramammarian findings such as erythema nodosum and/or arthritis are more common in pregnant women [22–26].

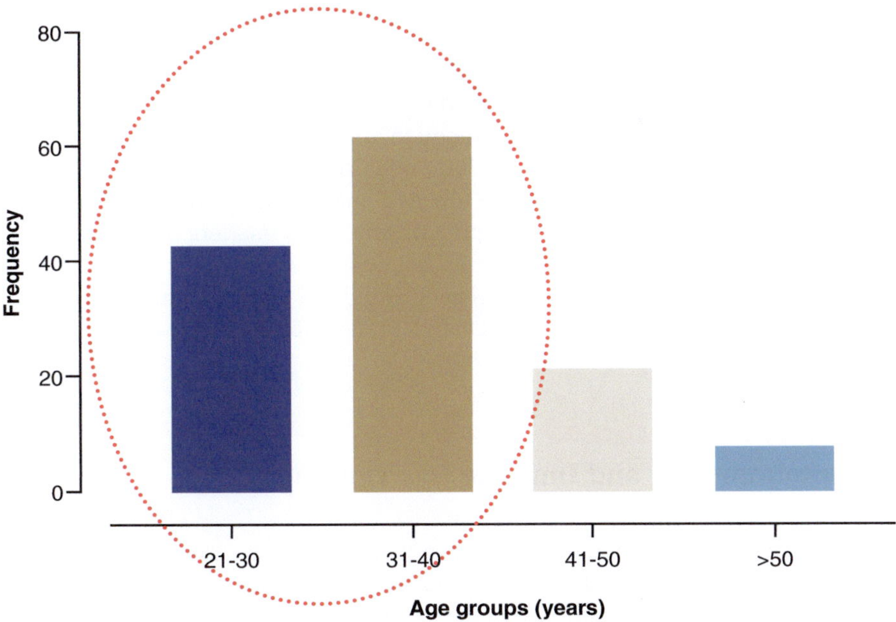

Fig. 1 Age distribution of our IGM patients

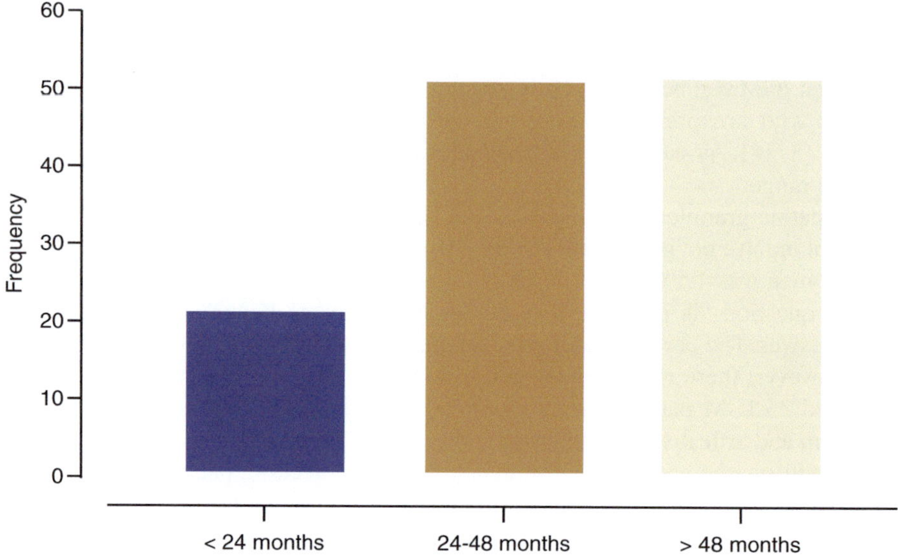

Fig. 2 Duration between the diagnosis and last birth in our IGM patients

Another factor in the etiology of IGM is breastfeeding at the time of diagnosis [1, 2]. There are two important points in breastfeeding: the breastfeeding history of the IGM patient and whether breastfeeding is present at the time of the diagnosis or not. Patients with IGM diagnosis before the reproductive age and, although rare, the fact that men may be diagnosed with IGM suggest that breastfeeding at the time of diagnosis has no direct role in IGM etiology [5, 18].

In our study [8], the time from the last childbirth to the diagnosis of IGM was investigated. The time periods were divided into three groups: <24 months, 24–48 months, and > 48 months. Approximately three quarters of patients were found to be diagnosed 24 months after the last delivery (Fig. 2).

As emphasized in the article, this brings highlight to the question: "Does breastfeeding prevent or delay the development of IGM, suggesting the possible contribution of autoimmunity/immune dysregulation?"

5 Autoimmunity and Immune Dysregulation

Recently, autoimmunity and immune dysregulation has been emphasized in the etiology of IGM. The arguments made are the use of immunosuppressive drugs such as corticosteroids and methotrexate in the treatment of IGM, the presence of common symptoms observed in rheumatological diseases such as erythema nodosum or arthritis, and coincidence with some rheumatological diseases such as Sjogren's syndrome and systemic lupus erythematosus [8, 27–33].

One of the first studies on this subject was by Erhan et al. [34]. The authors completed an immunohistochemical investigation of T and B lymphocytes in the specimen. A predominance of T cells was observed. In a similar study by Chen et al. [16], CD3-positive lymphocytes in the peripheral aggregation zone of neutrophils within granulomatous lesions were seen more than CD20-positive lymphocytes. In light of these findings, we compared the peripheral lymphocyte subgroups of IGM patients to investigate whether the change in T and B lymphocytes had a reflection in the peripheral blood [35]. We found that while IGM patients' T helper lymphocytes were lower than the control group, cytotoxic T lymphocytes and natural killer T cells were higher. All these findings may propound a possible immune dysregulation in IGM [36].

There are two cytokine studies in IGM [37, 38]. In our study, we found that levels of the interleukin-8, interleukin-10, and interleukin-17 were higher in patients with IGM than controls. We thought that interleukin-8 and interleukin-17, known as pro-inflammatory cytokines, had a role in the pathogenesis of IGM. High interleukin-10 levels especially in patients in remission reduced the release of proinflammatory cytokines as well as suppressed their function to control the inflammation in IGM [37]. Saydam et al. [38] found that levels of interleukin-22 and interleukin-33 were higher in IGM patients and concluded that these findings support the role of autoimmunity in the etiopathogenesis of IGM.

Autoantibodies have also been studied in patients with IGM. Ozel et al. [39] detected the rheumatoid factor in six of eight IGM patients, antinuclear antibody in two patients, and anti-double-stranded DNA positivity in two patients. In another study, they investigated antinuclear antibody and extractable nuclear antigen in patients with IGM [40]. However, they emphasized that their study did not support the autoimmune basis for IGM. In our study [41], we investigated the rheumatoid factor, antinuclear antibody, anti-double-stranded DNA antibody, anti-cyclic citrullinated peptide antibody, and perinuclear antineutrophil cytoplasmic antibody in IGM patients with active lesions, in remission, and in the control group. But our study did not support a positive clinical outcome of these autoantibodies in IGM.

An interesting finding is the seasonal fluctuations of IGM as highlighted in the epidemiology section [8, 42]. The fact that IGM is common especially in the spring and early days of summer brings to mind the question of whether IGM is an autoimmune disease triggered by viral infections.

In conclusion, all these findings suggest that immune dysregulation and autoimmunity play an important role in the etiopathogenesis of IGM.

References

1. Benson JR, Dumitru D. Idiopathic granulomatous mastitis: presentation, investigation and management. Future Oncol. 2016;12:1381–94. https://doi.org/10.2217/fon-2015-0038.
2. Yin Y, Liu X, Meng Q, Han X, Zhang H, Lv Y. Idiopathic granulomatous mastitis: etiology, clinical manifestation, diagnosis and treatment. J Investig Surg. 2022;35(3):709–20. https://doi.org/10.1080/08941939.2021.1894516.

3. Schelfout K, Tjalma WA, Cooremans ID, Coeman DC, Colpaert CG, Buytaert PM. Observations of an idiopathic granulomatous mastitis. Eur J Obstet Gynecol Reprod Biol. 2001;97:260–2. https://doi.org/10.1016/s0301-2115(00)00546-7.
4. Al-Khaffaf B, Knox F, Bundred NJ. Idiopathic granulomatous mastitis: a 25-year experience. J Am Coll Surg. 2008;206:269–73. https://doi.org/10.1016/j.jamcollsurg.2007.07.041.
5. Bani-Hani KE, Yaghan RJ, Matalka II, Shatnawi NJ. Idiopathic granulomatous mastitis: time to avoid unnecessary mastectomies. Breast J. 2004;10:318–22. https://doi.org/10.1111/j.1075-122X.2004.21336.x.
6. Baslaim MM, Khayat HA, Al-Amoudi SA. Idiopathic granulomatous mastitis: a heterogeneous disease with variable clinical presentation. World J Surg. 2007;31:1677–81. https://doi.org/10.1007/s00268-007-9116-1.
7. Gurleyik G, Aktekin A, Aker F, Karagulle H, Saglam A. Medical and surgical treatment of idiopathic granulomatous lobular mastitis: a benign inflammatory disease mimicking invasive carcinoma. J Breast Cancer. 2012;15:119–23. https://doi.org/10.4048/jbc.2012.15.1.119.
8. Koksal H. What are the new findings with regard to the mysterious disease idiopathic granulomatous mastitis? Surg Today. 2021;51:1158–68. https://doi.org/10.1007/s00595-020-02204-2.
9. Oran EŞ, Gurdal SO, Yankol Y, Öznur M, Calay Z, Tunacı M, et al. Management of idiopathic granulomatous mastitis diagnosed by core biopsy: a retrospective multicenter study. Breast J. 2013;19:411–8. https://doi.org/10.1111/tbj.12123.
10. Agrawal A, Pabolu S. A rare case of idiopathic granulomatous mastitis in a nulliparous woman with hyperprolactinemia. Cureus. 2019;11(5):e4680. https://doi.org/10.7759/cureus.4680.
11. Bellavia M, Damiano G, Palumbo VD, Spinelli G, Tomasello G, Marrazzo A, et al. Granulomatous mastitis during chronic antidepressant therapy: is it possible a conservative therapeutic approach? J Breast Cancer. 2012;15:371–2. https://doi.org/10.4048/jbc.2012.15.3.371.
12. Destek S, Gul VO, Ahioglu S, Serin KR. Pituitary adenoma and hyperprolactinemia accompanied by idiopathic granulomatous mastitis. Case Rep Endocrinol. 2017;2017:3974291. https://doi.org/10.1155/2017/3974291.
13. Holla S, Amberkar MB, Kamath A, Kamalkishore MK, Ommurugan B. Risperidone induced granulomatous mastitis secondary to hyperprolactinemia in a non-pregnant woman-a rare case report in a bipolar disorder. J Clin Diagn Res. 2017;11:FD01-FD03. https://doi.org/10.7860/JCDR/2017/20733.9278.
14. Li J, McGregor HP. Idiopathic granulomatous mastitis associated with hyperprolactinemia: a nonoperative approach. Breast J. 2017;23:742–4. https://doi.org/10.1111/tbj.12914.
15. Lin CH, Hsu CW, Tsao TY, Chou J. Idiopathic granulomatous mastitis associated with risperidone-induced hyperprolactinemia. Diagn Pathol. 2012;7:2. https://doi.org/10.1186/1746-1596-7-2.
16. Chen L, Zhang XY, Wang YW, Zhao QF, Ding HY. Granulomatous lobular mastitis: a clinicopathological analysis of 300 cases. Zhonghua Bing Li Xue Za Zhi. 2019;48:231–6. https://doi.org/10.3760/cma.j.issn.0529-5807.2019.03.012.
17. Colao A, Sarno AD, Cappabianca P, Briganti F, Pivonello R, Somma CD, et al. Gender differences in the prevalence, clinical features and response to cabergoline in hyperprolactinemia. Eur J Endocrinol. 2003;148:325–31. https://doi.org/10.1530/eje.0.1480325.
18. Yaghan RJ, Ayoub NM, Shenawi HM, Yaghan LR. Idiopathic granulomatous mastitis in the male population: a clinical analysis of 13 reported cases. Breast J. 2020;26:1481–2. https://doi.org/10.1111/tbj.13778.
19. Fahmy J, Halabi-Tawil M, Bagot M, Tournant B, Petit A. Erythema nodosum during the course of idiopathic granulomatous mastitis. Ann Dermatol Venereol. 2015;142:46–9. https://doi.org/10.1016/j.annder.2014.09.009.
20. Jacquin-Porretaz C, Devalland C, Delapparent T, Nardin C, Dupond AS. Idiopathic granulomatous mastitis associated with erythema nodosum. Ann Dermatol Venereol. 2019;146:571–6. https://doi.org/10.1016/j.annder.2019.04.023.

21. Uysal E, Soran A, Sezgin E, Granulomatous Mastitis Study Group. Factors related to recurrence of idiopathic granulomatous mastitis: what do we learn from a multicentre study? ANZ J Surg. 2018;88:635–9. https://doi.org/10.1111/ans.14115.
22. Sener Bahce Z, Aktas H. Patients with idiopathic granulomatous mastitis accompanied by erythema nodosum. Int J Clin Pract. 2021;75:e13928. https://doi.org/10.1111/ijcp.13928.
23. Garcia-Rodiguez JA, Pattullo A. Idiopathic granulomatous mastitis: a mimicking disease in a pregnant woman: a case report. BMC Res Notes. 2013;6:95. https://doi.org/10.1186/1756-0500-6-95.
24. Kornfeld HW, Mitchell KB. Management of idiopathic granulomatous mastitis in lactation: case report and review of the literature. Int Breastfeed J. 2021;16:23. https://doi.org/10.1186/s13006-021-00370-8.
25. Lucas R, Gussman D, Polis RL, Rattigan MI, Matulewicz TJ. Idiopathic granulomatous mastitis with erythema nodosum simulating breast abscess in pregnancy: a case report. Obstet Med. 2014;7:37–9. https://doi.org/10.1177/1753495X13502474.
26. Salesi M, Karimifar M, Salimi F, Mahzouni P. A case of granulomatous mastitis with erythema nodosum and arthritis. Rheumatol Int. 2011;31:1093–5. https://doi.org/10.1007/s00296-009-1273-0.
27. Godazandeh G, Shojaee L, Alizadeh-Navaei R, Hessami A. Corticosteroids in idiopathic granulomatous mastitis: a systematic review and meta-analysis. Surg Today. 2021;51:1897–905. https://doi.org/10.1007/s00595-021-02234-4.
28. Haddad M, Sheybani F, Arian M, Gharib M. Methotrexate-based regimen as initial treatment of patients with idiopathic granulomatous mastitis. Breast J. 2020;26:325–7. https://doi.org/10.1111/tbj.13590.
29. Kehribar DY, Duran TI, Polat AK, Ozgen M. Effectiveness of methotrexate in idiopathic granulomatous mastitis treatment. Am J Med Sci. 2020;360:560–5. https://doi.org/10.1016/j.amjms.2020.05.029.
30. Letourneux C, Diemunsch P, Korganow AS, Akladios CY, Bellocq JP, Mathelin C. First report of granulomatous mastitis associated with Sjögren's syndrome. World J Surg Oncol. 2013;11:268. https://doi.org/10.1186/1477-7819-11-268.
31. Papila Kundaktepe B, Velidedeoğlu M, Mete B. The effect of methotrexate monotherapy on treatment-resistant idiopathic granulomatous mastitis patients. Surgeon. 2021;20:e13–9. S1479-666X(21)00065-2
32. Postolova A, Troxell ML, Wapnir IL, Genovese MC. Methotrexate in the treatment of idiopathic granulomatous mastitis. J Rheumatol. 2020;47:924–7. https://doi.org/10.3899/jrheum.181205.
33. Yazigi G, Trieu BH, Landis M, Parikh JG, Mangal M. Granulomatous mastitis: a rare case with Sjogren's syndrome and complications. Cureus. 2019;11:e5359. https://doi.org/10.7759/cureus.5359.
34. Erhan Y, Veral A, Kara E, Ozdemir N, Kapkac M, Ozdedeli E, et al. A clinicopathologic study of a rare clinical entity mimicking breast carcinoma: idiopathic granulomatous mastitis. Breast. 2000;9:52–6. https://doi.org/10.1054/brst.1999.0072.
35. Emsen A, Koksal H, Ozdemir H, Kadoglou N, Artac H. The alteration of lymphocyte subsets in idiopathic granulomatous mastitis. Turk J Med Sci. 2021;51:1905–11. https://doi.org/10.3906/sag-2012-192.
36. Ucaryilmaz H, Koksal H, Emsen A, Kadoglou N, Dixon JM, Artac H. The role of regulatory T and B cells in the etiopathogenesis of idiopathic granulomatous mastitis. Immunol Investig. 2022;51:357–67. https://doi.org/10.1080/08820139.2020.1832114.
37. Koksal H, Vatansev H, Artac H, Kadoglou N. The clinical value of interleukins-8, −10, and −17 in idiopathic granulomatous mastitis. Clin Rheumatol. 2020;39:1671–7. https://doi.org/10.1007/s10067-020-04925-8.
38. Saydam M, Yilmaz KB, Sahin M, Yanik H, Akinci M, Yilmaz I, et al. New findings on autoimmune etiology of idiopathic granulomatous mastitis: serum IL-17, IL-22 and IL-23 levels of patients. J Investig Surg. 2020;34:993–7. https://doi.org/10.1080/08941939.2020.1725190.

39. Ozel L, Unal A, Unal E, Kara M, Erdoğdu E, Krand O, et al. Granulomatous mastitis: is it an autoimmune disease? Diagnostic and therapeutic dilemmas. Surg Today. 2012;42:729–33. https://doi.org/10.1007/s00595-011-0046-z.
40. Altintoprak F, Karakece E, Kivilcim T, Dikicier E, Cakmak G, Celebi F, et al. Idiopathic granulomatous mastitis: an autoimmune disease? Sci World J. 2013;2013:148727. https://doi.org/10.1155/2013/148727.
41. Koksal H. The clinical utility of autoantibodies in patients with idiopathic granulomatous mastitis. J Invest Surg. 2022;35:325–9. https://doi.org/10.1080/08941939.2020.1861666.
42. Tekin L, Dinç Elibol F. Is there any relationship between granulomatous mastitis and seasons? An analysis of seasonal frequency, clinical, and radiologic findings. Eur J Breast Health. 2020;16:235–43. https://doi.org/10.5152/ejbh.2020.5897.

The Role of Genetic Factors

Leyla Ozer ⓘ

Many possible causes of idiopathic granulomatous mastitis (IGM) are thought to have a role in the formation of the disease. Several factors (autoimmunity, infections, hormonal abnormalities, breast trauma, and obesity) are blamed for the etiology of IGM [1, 2]. Autoimmune-mediated inflammatory response stands out among the possible mechanisms. Altintoprak et al. [1] hypothesized that ethnical differences and autoimmune responses are the main mechanisms of IGM [2]. In this review they searched articles related with IGM and they noticed that the patients originated from certain ethnic groups. In a literature search between 1995 and 2014, they found that the cases were frequently reported from Mediterranean and Asian countries [2]. The largest case series of IGM patients were reported in Iran (374 patients) and Turkey (>200 patients), respectively [2, 3]. The significant relationship between a particular ethnic group and the frequency of disease suggests that genetic differences between individuals may have an important role in the susceptibility to the disease. The underlying genetic causes are not fully understood and a limited number of studies were reported on genetic causes; however, genetic variations and gene expression changes potentially may be involved in causative factors.

1 Genetic Polymorphism Studies

In recent years, several studies have been reported analyzing the relationship between IGM susceptibility and the presence of certain types of genetic polymorphisms. Identification of SNPs (single-nucleotide polymorphisms) can help us to

L. Ozer (✉)
Department of Medical Genetics, Faculty of Medicine, Yuksek Ihtisas University, Ankara, Türkiye

Microgen Genetic Diagnostic Centers, Ankara, Türkiye

understand the genetic basis of complex diseases. Bercot et al. [4] reported a case with granulomatous mastitis caused by *Corynebacterium kroppenstedtii* infection. They showed disrupted NOD2 protein (nucleotide-binding oligomerization domain-containing protein 2) function and the NOD2 gene sequencing revealed an SNP variant of the NOD2 gene (SNP13 Leu1007fsinsC) [4]. The SNP13 Leu1007fsinsC variant was reported as one of the most frequently observed polymorphisms in patients with Crohn's disease [4]. NOD2 plays an important role in the immune response. The NOD2 protein shows a significantly elevated level of expression in the peripheral blood leukocytes. It recognizes molecules containing muramyl dipeptide (MDP) which is found in some bacteria and which stimulates an immune reaction. Binding of NOD2 to its ligand stimulates the production and release of cytokines by activating the NF-κB protein. NOD2 also regulates processes like cell differentiation, proliferation, and apoptosis by activating the mitogen-activated protein kinase (MAPK) signaling pathway [5].

Some of the studies focused on common genetic polymorphisms such as MTHFR and ACE gene polymorphisms. Lei et al. [6] investigated the relationship between IGM and methylene tetrahydrofolate reductase (MTHFR) gene polymorphism (C677T and A1298C). They studied 55 IGM patients and found a significant relationship with C677T polymorphisms. The authors hypothesized that MTHFR C677T may have a role in the formation of idiopathic granulomatous mastitis. Destek et al. [7] also studied gene polymorphisms in a patient with IGM and they found the presence of MTHFR-C 677 TT, β-fibrinogen-455G/A, PA'I-1 5 G/5 G, and ACE 'I/D gene polymorphisms.

The human leukocyte antigen (HLA) region or complex localizes on chromosome 6 and includes several immune response genes. The HLA region is composed of 252 genes with different polymorphisms, which is the largest number of polymorphism within the genome. Human leukocyte antigen (HLA) genes are found to be associated with autoimmune disorders. The first known HLA association study on IGM was reported by Koksal [8]. Forty-eight IGM patients were compared with healthy controls in terms of HLA gene polymorphisms. The author observed that the prevalence of HLA-A * 10, HLA-A * 2403, HLA-B * 18, and HLA-DR * 17 were higher in IGM patients compared to the control group, whilst the prevalence of HLA-A * 29, HLA-B * 14, and HLA-DR * 1 were lower. The author hypothesized that increased incidence of both HLA-A*2403 and HLA-B*18 antigens may be related to the humoral immunity and autoimmunity in IGM pathogenesis [8]. Although the results of this study are valuable, it will be more meaningful with the increase in HLA association studies in IGM patients from different geographic regions and different ethnic groups.

Genome-wide association studies (GWAS) are used in genetic studies to identify inherited genetic risk variants associated with relevant diseases especially complex diseases. Although GWAS in autoimmune diseases and infectious diseases were reported, GWAS related to infectious mastitis were reported in animals, and according to the studies, DCK, SLC4A4, and EDN3 genes may play a role in response to pathogens. However, no GWAS related to IGM was found in literature [9].

Schelfout et al. [9] postulated that there might be a relationship between IGM and α1-antitrypsin (AAT) deficiency [10]. The authors reported the presence of IGM in a case of α1-antitrypsin deficiency. α1-Antitrypsin deficiency is a genetic disorder caused by SERPINA gene mutations. The primary function of AAT protein is to protect tissues from the harmful effects of proteases secreted by active neutrophils. Patients with AAT deficiency have risks of hepatic dysfunction, chronic obstructive lung disease (emphysema and/or bronchiectasis), panniculitis, and C-ANCA-positive vasculitis. They postulated that AAT deficiency may cause IGM but this was only reported in one patient and further studies should be designed to investigate SERPINA1 gene variations in IGM patients [10].

2 Gene Expression Studies

A limited number of gene expression studies were reported. Zhu et al. [11] designed a study to identify gene expression profiles of idiopathic granulomatous mastitis. They compared the differences between biopsy materials of granulomatous tissue and normal tissue in terms of differentially expressed RNAs. Gene expression analysis focused on immune system genes to enlighten the underlying immune mechanism and breast cancer genes to show the difference and relationship between IGM and breast cancer. Whole gene expression profiles detected 136 upregulated and 71 downregulated mRNAs between the IGM tissues and control tissues. In the study, DNAJC27-AS1 was reported as the highest unregulated mRNA and TRAV12-1 as the lowest downregulated mRNA. Although prednisone has been commonly used in the treatment of IGM; HSD11B1 mRNA, which was the drug target of prednisone, had lower expression in IGM tissues [11]. However, several studies demonstrated that prednisone treatment has an effective role in medical treatment at reducing the size and extent of the lesion and the recurrence risk. RNA-sequencing differential expression analysis revealed that the detected differentially expressed mRNAs take a significant part in the immune system. They compared gene expression profiles of two groups (IGM tissues and normal tissue) to define the gene-gene interaction related with IGM. The mRNAs related with immune system were classified into two groups: network A and B. Network A includes FCGR1A, TRIM29, GBP1, GBP5, LILRB4, HCK, C1QB, SLC7A7, IGSF6, and CD79A genes and network B includes TCN1, MMP9, TNFAIP6, CHIT1, LYZ, SLPI, CHI3L1, CTSC, PIGR, and MMP12 genes [11]. The hub gene (gene with high correlation in candidate modules) of network A was the FCGR1A gene which was associated with IgG and protein binding. The TCN1 was the hub gene in network B that was associated with cobalamin binding. FCGR1A is the drug target of methyl aminolevulinate, and TCN1 is the drug target of hydroxycobalamin [10]. These two networks contain immune system-related genes and represent the possible role of immune mechanisms in the pathogenesis of IGM. When the authors analyzed the gene expression profiles of breast cancer, they found that 73.6% of IGM gene expressions were high in both breast cancer and IGM tissues. According to the results of the study, they concluded that

IGM etiology is due to immune system dysfunction and they found a similarity between breast cancer and IGM in some previous studies [11].

Another gene expression study was reported by Aksan et al. [12]. Their study aimed to investigate the miR-155, let-7c, miR-21, and PTEN levels of patients with IGM and breast cancer [12]. MicroRNA (miRNA) is a short noncoding RNA molecule which has a role in gene silencing and the regulation of gene expression. In recent years, miRNAs have been accepted as a potential biomarker. Several studies have reported the use of miRNAs in the diagnosis of diseases. In the Aksan's study [12], the authors chose to analyze miR-21, miR-155, and let-7c levels because in previous studies, miR-21, miR-155, and let-7c expressions were used as potential biomarkers of breast cancer [11]. They also studied the PTEN expression levels due to the negative regulation of PTEN gene expression by miR-21. According to the results of this study, the authors concluded that miR-21 may be a potential biomarker for breast cancer in the differential diagnosis of IGM. They also found a negative correlation between miR-21 and PTEN in breast cancer. It was observed that miR-21 was overexpressed whilst PTEN expression decreased in breast cancer. MiR-21 expression and PTEN levels were concluded to be useful biomarkers in the differential diagnosis of IGM and breast cancer [12].

3 Human Microbiome Studies

Commensal and symbiotic microorganisms can be found in the human body. The microbiome includes the genome of microorganisms and their ecosystems. Environmental factors, nutrition habits, and host genetics may affect the occurrence of the wide microbial diversity. The microbiome and microbial products may have a role in the regulation of immune response in the host. The interaction between the human microbiome and immune system plays an important role in the etiopathogenesis of several diseases. Recently, several studies have concentrated on the role of the microbiome in the pathogenesis of autoimmune diseases [12]. With rapid developments in sequencing technology and bioinformatics methods, the number of metagenomic studies has increased. Clarifying the effect of the human microbiome on the host immune system enables the development of new therapeutic approaches. There are numerous studies investigating the relationship between intestinal microbiome and autoimmune diseases [13, 14]. The gut microbiome is composed of millions of microbes, and it plays a crucial role in host immunity and metabolism. Several studies have been reported to analyze the gut microbiome in autoimmune diseases, such as systemic lupus erythematosus, inflammatory bowel disease, multiple sclerosis, rheumatoid arthritis, and type 1 diabetes but not in granulomatous mastitis [13, 14].

The microflora of IGM is still incompletely defined. The number of studies aimed to characterize the microbiome in IGM is very limited. The first study to use next-generation sequencing in this field was conducted by Yu et al. [15]. They studied the microbiome analysis of breast tissue in IGM patients and found

Corynebacterium in all patients (19/19). *Corynebacterium* was the most abundant taxon in 40% of patients. *Corynebacterium kroppenstedtii* is the predominant *Corynebacterium* species in these patients (11/19) [15]. Previous studies support Yu et al.'s [15] finding that *Corynebacterium*, especially *C. kroppenstedtii*, was commonly detected in IGM patients. Another study profiling the microbiota of IGM patients revealed that *Pseudomonas*, *Brevundimonas*, *Stenotrophomonas*, *Acinetobacter*, and *Aspergillus* were the most detected pathogens. In contrast to previous studies, *C. kroppenstedtii* was not the predominant pathogen of IGM patients according to this study [16]. Metagenomic studies with NGS technology are considered as a potential powerful technique to detect pathogenic microorganisms in the pathogenesis of granulomatous mastitis. Metagenomics will expand our knowledge regarding the microbial diagnosis of IGM and in order to find new treatment options, but further studies are needed due to the limited number of metagenomics studies on IGM.

4 The Future

Very little is known about genetic risk factors of IGM. With the rapid development of genetic technologies, studies reporting the detection of genetic factors that play a role in the formation of various diseases have attracted great interest. New investigations will be necessary to define the genetic factors in IGM susceptibility. Further genetic studies are required to discover the granulomatous mastitis risk loci and the role of microbiota in the pathogenesis of IGM.

References

1. Altintoprak F, Kivilcim T, Ozkan OV. Aetiology of idiopathic granulomatous mastitis. World J Clin Cases. 2014;2:852–8. https://doi.org/10.12998/wjcc.v2.i12.852.
2. Wolfrum A, Kümmel S, Theuerkauf I, Pelz E, Reinisch M. Granulomatous mastitis: a therapeutic and diagnostic challenge. Breast Care (Basel). 2018;13:413–8. https://doi.org/10.1159/000495146.
3. Kaviani A, Vasigh M, Omranipour R, Mahmoudzadeh H, Elahi A, Farivar L, et al. Idiopathic granulomatous mastitis: looking for the most effective therapy with the least side effects according to the severity of the disease in 374 patients in Iran. Breast J. 2019;25:672–7. https://doi.org/10.1111/tbj.13300.
4. Bercot B, Kannengiesser C, Oudin C, Grandchamp B, Sanson-le Pors MJ, Mouly S, et al. First description of NOD2 variant associated with defective neutrophil responses in a woman with granulomatous mastitis related to corynebacteria. J Clin Microbiol. 2009;47:3034–7. https://doi.org/10.1128/JCM.00561-09.
5. Negroni A, Pierdomenico M, Cucchiara S, Stronati L. NOD2 and inflammation: current insights. J Inflamm Res. 2018;11:49–60. https://doi.org/10.2147/JIR.S137606.
6. Lei QR, Yang X, Miao CM, Wang JC, Yang Y. Relationship between granulomatous lobular mastitis and methylene tetrahydrofolate reductase gene polymorphism. World J Clin Cases. 2020;8:4017–21. https://doi.org/10.12998/wjcc.v8.i18.4017.

7. Destek S, Gul VO, Ahioglu S. A variety of gene polymorphisms associated with idiopathic granulomatous mastitis. J Surg Case Rep. 2016;rjw156 https://doi.org/10.1093/jscr/rjw156.

8. Koksal H. Human leukocyte antigens class I and II in patients with idiopathic granulomatous mastitis. Am J Surg. 2019;218:605–8. https://doi.org/10.1016/j.amjsurg.2019.01.038.

9. Schelfout K, Tjalma WA, Cooremans ID, Coeman DC, Colpaert CG, Buytaert PM. Observations of an idiopathic granulomatous mastitis. Eur J Obstet Gynecol Reprod Biol. 2001;97:260–2. https://doi.org/10.2147/JIR.S137606.

10. Mozzi A, Pontremoli C, Sironi M. Genetic susceptibility to infectious diseases: current status and future perspectives from genome-wide approaches. Infect Genet Evol. 2018;66:286–307. https://doi.org/10.1016/j.meegid.2017.09.028.

11. Zhu Q, Wang L, Wang P. The identification of gene expression profiles associated with granulomatous mastitis. Breast Care. 2020;16:319–27. https://doi.org/10.1159/000507474.

12. Aksan H, Kundaktepe BP, Sayili U, Velidedeoglu M, Simsek G, Koksal S, et al. Circulating miR-155, let-7c, miR-21, and PTEN levels in differential diagnosis and prognosis of idiopathic granulomatous mastitis and breast cancer. Biofactors. 2020;46:955–62. https://doi.org/10.1002/biof.1676.

13. Gundogdu A, Nalbantoglu U. Human genome-microbiome interaction: metagenomics frontiers for the aetiopathology of autoimmune diseases. Microb Genom. 2017;3:e000112. https://doi.org/10.1099/mgen.0.000112.

14. Volkova A, Ruggles K. Predictive metagenomic analysis of autoimmune disease identifies robust autoimmunity and disease specific microbial signatures. Biorvix. 2020; https://doi.org/10.1101/779967.

15. Yu HJ, Deng H, Ma J, Huang SJ, Yang JM, Huang YF, et al. Clinical metagenomic analysis of bacterial communities in breast abscesses of granulomatous mastitis. Int J Infect Dis. 2016;53:30–3. https://doi.org/10.1016/j.ijid.2016.10.015.

16. Wang J, Xu H, Li Z, Li F, Yang Y, Yu X, et al. Pathogens in patients with granulomatous lobular mastitis. Int J Infect Dis. 2019;81:123–7. https://doi.org/10.1016/j.ijid.2019.01.034.

Clinical Manifestations and Classification

Hande Koksal ⓘ

Although IGM generally presents with local symptoms and signs in one breast, it can occur bilaterally. There may also be rarely extramammarian manifestations including erythema nodosum and arthritis. The most common symptoms or signs of IGM are mass, redness, and pain. Symptoms and signs of IGM can be seen in Table 1 [1, 2].

Table 1 The symptoms and signs of 134 patients with idiopathic granulomatous mastitis [2]

	Manifestations	n (%)
Local manifestation	Mass	129 (96.3)
	Pain	120 (89.6)
	Erythema	91 (67.9)
	Abscess	77 (57.5)
	Axillary lymphadenopathy	41 (30.6)
	Nipple retraction	14 (10.4)
	Ulcer	13 (9.7)
	Fistula	11 (8.3)
	Peau d'orange	10 (7.5)
	Nipple discharge	4 (3)
Extramammarian manifestations	Erythema nodosum	7 (5.2)
	Arthritis	3 (2.2)
	Episcleritis*	

*Episcleritis has been reported only as a case report [3]

H. Koksal (✉)
Department of General Surgery, Selcuk University, Faculty of Medicine, Konya, Türkiye

© The Author(s), under exclusive license to Springer Nature Switzerland AG 2023
H. Koksal, N. Kadoglou (eds.), *Idiopathic Granulomatous Mastitis*,
https://doi.org/10.1007/978-3-031-30391-3_5

1   Local Manifestations

Mass is the symptom and sign met in majority of patients with IGM (96.3%). It is usually present in a single breast and can be seen in any quadrant of the breast (Fig. 1). However, it is slightly more common in the upper outer quadrant or sub-areolar region. The mass is generally firm and ill-defined on physical examination. It may also be accompanied by tenderness, erythema, or other local manifestations [1, 4, 5]. Mass sizes can reach up to 10 cm [6].

  Pain is one of the common complaints of IGM patients. The incidence of pain is variable in IGM patients (90% to 100%) [1, 2, 7, 8]. Inflammation is the body's defensive response to any harmful agent to which it is exposed in order to protect itself. Host cells (including immune system cells), blood vessels, proteins, and mediators play an important role in this highly complex response. The cardinal signs of inflammation are heat, redness, swelling, pain, and loss of function (Figs. 2,

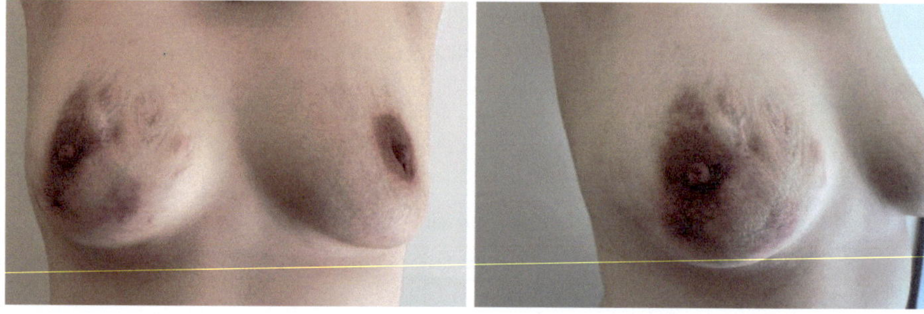

Fig. 1 A 31-year-old woman with a mass in the lower inner quadrant of the right breast and skin changes due to a previous abscess

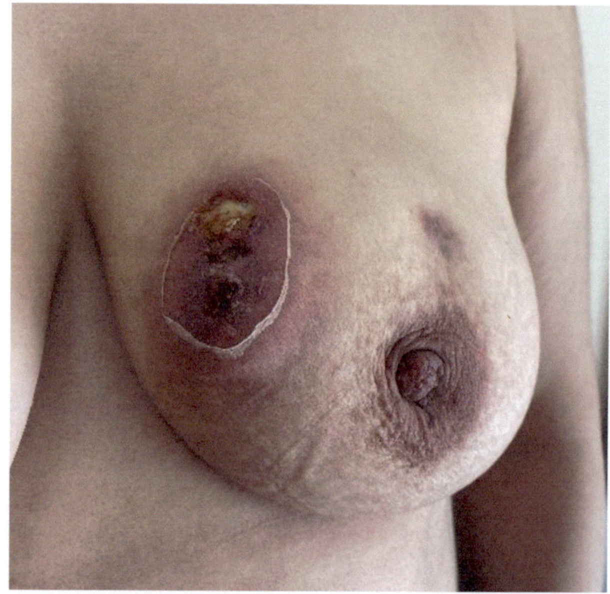

Fig. 2 A 33-year-old woman with an ulcerated mass and erythema in the upper inner quadrant of the left breast. Nipple retraction is also evident

3, and 4). Therefore, pain experienced by the patient may be a sign of inflammation. In inflammation, some mediators such as prostaglandins and bradykinin cause pain [9].

Erythema is another important symptom and sign of IGM [1, 2, 7, 8]. The possible cause of erythema in IGM is inflammation (Fig. 5). During the inflammatory process, after temporary vasoconstriction, arteriolar vasodilation occurs which leads to an increase in local blood flow in capillaries. All of these developments

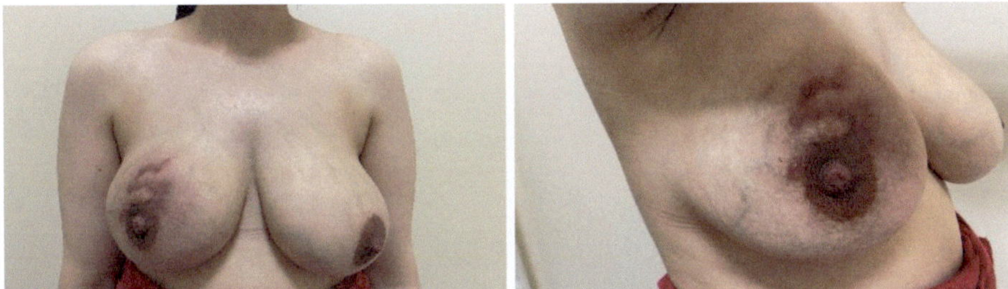

Fig. 3 A 29-year-old woman with IGM in the right breast. Skin changes after the treatment of the active lesion is notable

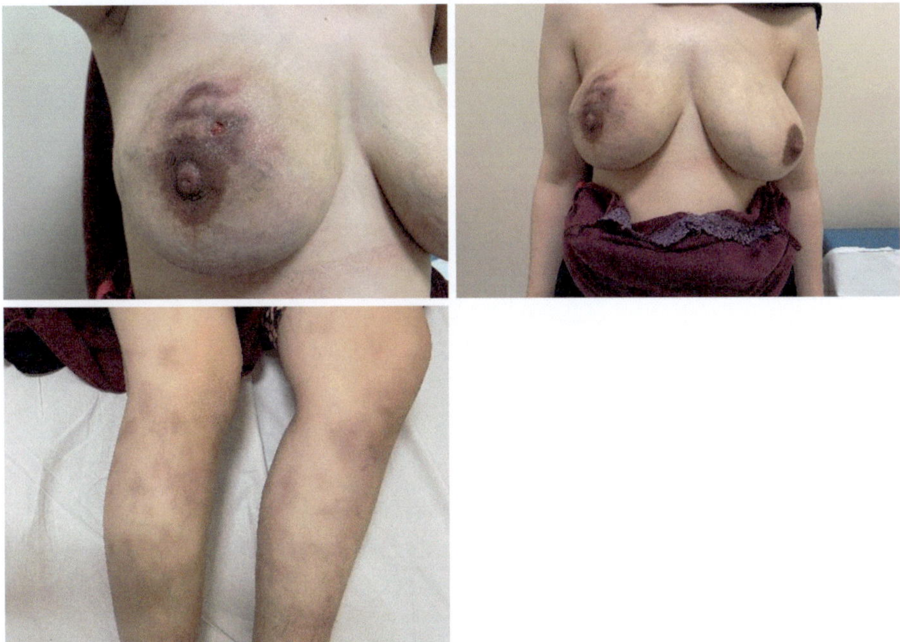

Fig. 4 A 28-year-old pregnant woman diagnosed with IGM in the right breast, fistula formation, and bilateral erythema nodosum on the lower extremities. She was treated by intralesional steroid injections till delivery, and then systemic steroid treatment was initiated

result in redness and increased local temperature, which are two important cardinal signs of inflammation [9].

Peau d'orange received its name due to its resemblance of an orange peel. The cause of peau d'orange is cutaneous lymphatic edema at Cooper's ligaments between the mammary gland and the skin [10]. The most common causes are inflammatory breast carcinoma, pseudoxanthoma elasticum, elephantiasis, and myxedema of Graves' disease. Rarely, it can also be seen in a chronic abscess as in IGM (Fig. 6).

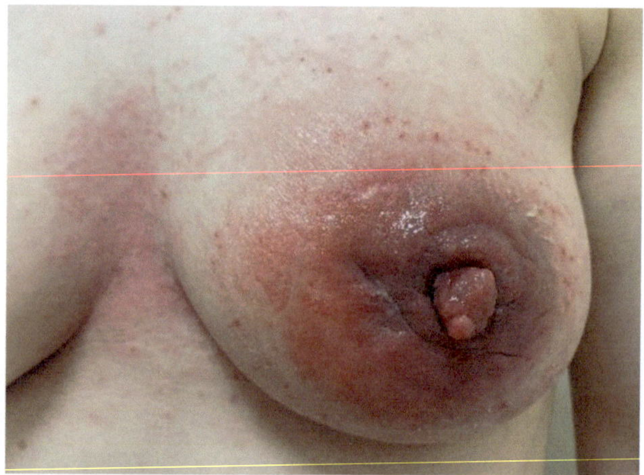

Fig. 5 Erythema and inflammation of the skin due to IGM in a 27-year-old woman

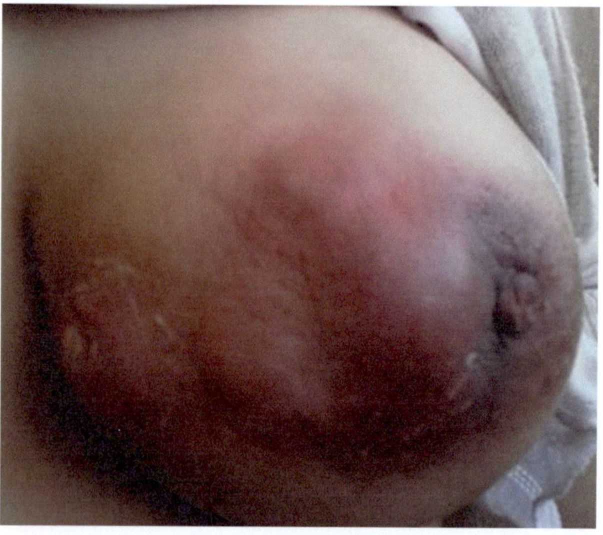

Fig. 6 An IGM patient with mass and erythema. Notice peau d'orange on the inner quadrants of the left breast

2   Extramammarian Manifestations

Extramammarian manifestations in IGM are erythema nodosum, arthritis, and episcleritis. The incidence of erythema nodosum or arthritis is 7.4–15.7% in IGM [2, 11].

Erythema nodosum, a variant of panniculitis, generally presents with eruption of erythematous tender nodules and plaques. They are more common in young women and often appear on the extensor aspects of the lower extremities [12–14]. Known etiologic factors of erythema nodosum include bacterial, viral, fungal, and protozoal infections, certain drugs, malignant diseases, autoimmune diseases, and rheumatologic diseases. However, in some patients the etiologic factors cannot be determined [13].

Erythema nodosum is one of the most common extramammarian findings of IGM (Figs. 4, 7, and 8). The frequency of erythema nodosum in IGM ranges from

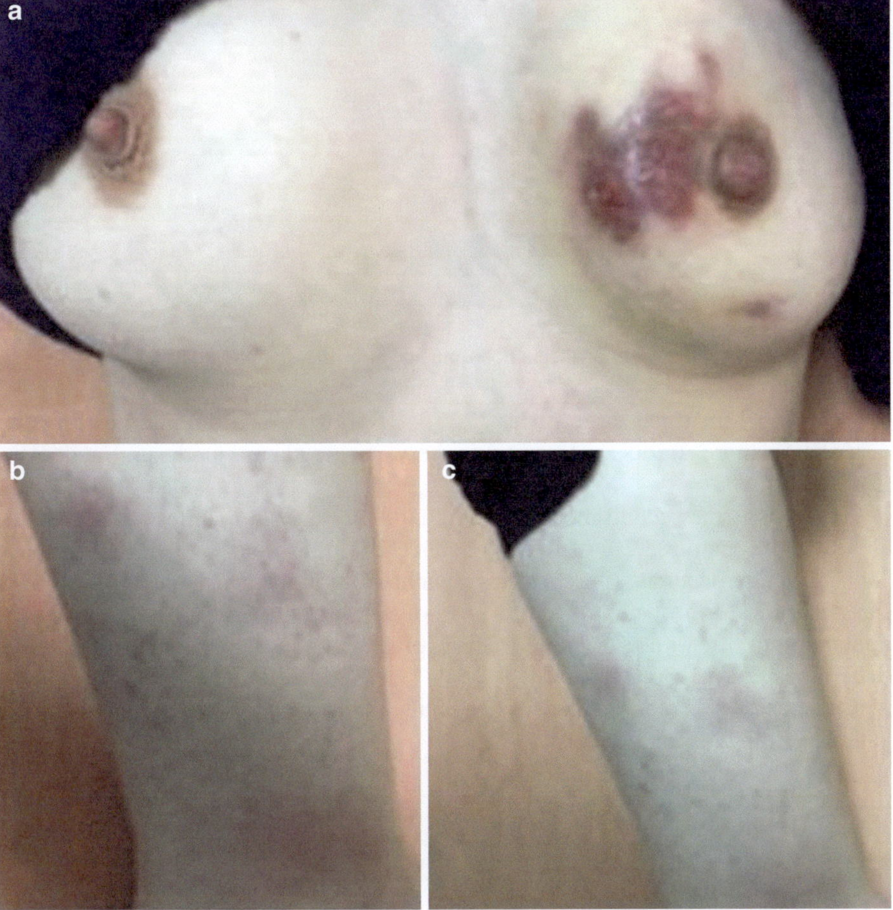

Fig. 7 The IGM patient with erythema nodosum on legs

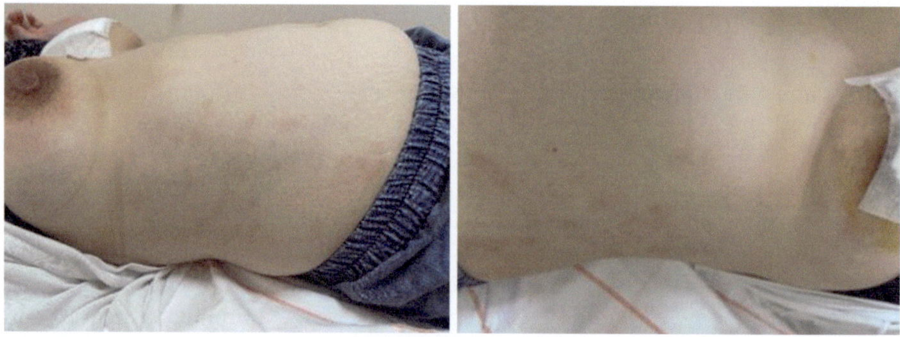

Fig. 8 A 44-year-old woman with a diagnosis of IGM on the left breast. The erythema nodosum lesions on her body started to heal after systemic steroid treatment

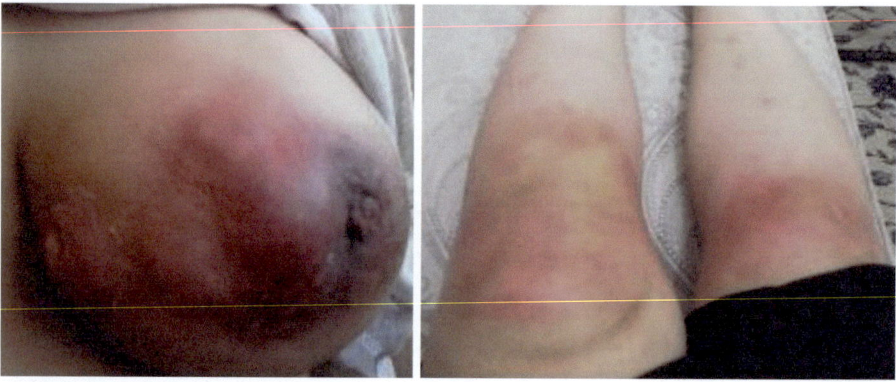

Fig. 9 The IGM patients with erythema nodosum and arthritis

4.4% to 6.6% in three large series [2, 15, 16]. However, multiple case reports describe a more frequent association between erythema nodosum and IGM [3, 17–39].

Arthritis is the second most common extramammarian manifestation of IGM, and it can be seen in 2.2% of IGM patients (Fig. 9). Similarly, to erythema nodosum, it can also occur at different times (synchronous or metachronous) [2]. Arthritis can be in the form of mono-, oligo-, or polyarthritis. It can also be unilateral or bilateral, and often knee or ankle joint involvement can be observed in the lower extremities [20, 22, 36, 37, 39].

Episcleritis was reported in only one patient as an accompanying finding and the pathophysiology is unknown [3].

3 Classification

Patients with IGM have very heterogeneous manifestations. While some patients only have a small, non-tender mass, some may have a mass with erythema, and some may have an abscess-like appearance covering nearly the entire breast. This heterogeneity may cause difficulties both in diagnosis and especially in determining an ideal treatment approach. Therefore, a classification is needed to determine an optimum treatment plan for these patients. There are three classifications suggested in the literature [16, 40–42].

Irkorucu [40, 41] proposes a classification for granulomatous mastitis. This proposed classification is shown in Table 2.

Yaghan et al. [16] proposed a classification considering the clinical findings of patients with IGM (Table 3).

These two classifications are very similar to each other. Interesting findings are high frequency of the pattern B in Jordan (nearly 53%) and pattern C (nearly 48%) in Turkey [2, 16]. It raises the question of whether there is a relationship between pattern type and ethnicity.

Another classification is proposed by Kaviani and Vasigh [42] which differently includes extramammarian manifestations as a separate title that suggests a systemic disease rather than a surgical entity (Table 4).

Although all these classification systems are based on clinical findings and have advantages and disadvantages on their own, the classification system proposed by

Table 2 Irkorucu's classification for all granulomatous mastitis

Types	Features
I	Limited superficial mastitis without abscess
II	Mastitis with only abscess formation
III	Mastitis with skin ulceration and fistulae
IV	Complex mastitis with painful mass, skin ulceration, abscess, and fistulae in one or two breasts
V	Mastitis with secondary complication of tuberculosis, sarcoidosis, syphilis, foreign body reaction, vasculitis, fungal and parasitic infections, etc.

Table 3 Clinically based classification for IGM [16]

Patterns	Features
A	Only mass
B	Pain and inflammation signs in addition to the mass
C	Abscess-like
D	Ulcer, sinus, or fistula in addition to the mass

Table 4 The classification of IGM [42]

Grade	Inflammatory	Soft tissue	Cutaneous lesions	Extramammary findings
I	Mild	Mild	−	−
II	Mild to moderate	Moderate to severe	−	−
III	Severe	Moderate to severe	+	−
IV	+/−	+/−	+/−	+

Irkorucu is the most detailed one. Kaviani and Vasigh's system has the subtitle of extramammarian manifestations, and therefore, this classification is important in terms of suggesting a systemic disease which may lead to a more appropriate treatment. A proper classification of the findings in this mysterious entity is essential in order to improve patients' outcomes.

References

1. Benson JR, Dumitru D. Idiopathic granulomatous mastitis: presentation, investigation and management. Future Oncol. 2016;12:1381–94. https://doi.org/10.2217/fon-2015-0038.
2. Koksal H. What are the new findings in mysterious disease: idiopathic granulomatous mastitis? Surg Today. 2021;51:1158–68. https://doi.org/10.1007/s00595-020-02204-2.
3. Pouchot J, Damade R, Barge J, Gaudin H, Vinceneux P. Idiopathic granulomatous mastitis and extramammary manifestations. Arch Pathol Lab Med. 1995;119:680.
4. Kiyak G, Dumlu EG, Kilinc I, Tokaç M, Akbaba S, Gurer A, et al. Management of idiopathic granulomatous mastitis: dilemmas in diagnosis and treatment. BMC Surg. 2014;4(14):66. https://doi.org/10.1186/1471-2482-14-66.
5. Naraynsingh V, Hariharan S, Dan D, Harnarayan P, Teelucksingh S. Conservative management for idiopathic granulomatous mastitis mimicking carcinoma: case reports and literature review. Breast Dis. 2010;31:57–60. https://doi.org/10.3233/BD-2009-0294.
6. Co M, Cheng VCC, Wei J, Wong SCY, Chan SMS, Shek T, et al. Idiopathic granulomatous mastitis: a 10-year study from a multicentre clinical database. Pathology. 2018;50:742–7. https://doi.org/10.1016/j.pathol.2018.08.010.
7. Steuer AB, Stern MJ, Cobos G, Castilla C, et al. Clinical characteristics and medical management of idiopathic granulomatous mastitis. JAMA Dermatol. 2020;156:460–4.
8. Tekin L, Dinç Elibol F. Is there any relationship between granulomatous mastitis and seasons? An analysis of seasonal frequency, clinical, and radiologic findings. Eur J Breast Health. 2020;16:235–43. https://doi.org/10.5152/ejbh.2020.5897.
9. Kumar V, Abbas A, Aster J. Inflammation and repair. In: Kumar V, Abbas A, Aster J, editors. Robbins basic pathology. 9th ed. Philadelphia: Elsevier; 2012. p. 29–73.
10. Bumin O, Bumin C. Meme. In: Bumin O, Bumin C, editors. Cerrahide Muayene Usulleri ve Hastalıklardaki Bulgular. 13th ed. Ankara: Türkiye Klinikleri Yayınevi; 1993. p. 115–24.
11. Chen L, Zhang XY, Wang YW, Zhao QF, Ding HY. Granulomatous lobular mastitis: a clinicopathological analysis of 300 cases. Zhonghua Bing Li Xue Za Zhi. 2019;48:231–6. https://doi.org/.3760/cma.j.issn.0529-5807.2019.03.012
12. Mana J, Marcoval J. Erythema nodosum. Clin Dermatol. 2007;25:288–94. https://doi.org/10.1016/j.clindermatol.2007.03.006.
13. Requena L, Yus ES. Erythema nodosum. Dermatol Clin. 2008;26:425–38. https://doi.org/10.1016/j.det.2008.05.014.
14. Schwartz RA, Nervi SJ. Erythema nodosum: a sign of systemic disease. Am Fam Physician. 2007;75:695–700.

15. Cetin K, Sikar HE, Gulluoglu BM. Idiopathic granulomatous mastitis with erythema nodosum: is it a variant of clinical presentation indicating treatment resistance? A retrospective cohort study. Breast J. 2020;26:1645–51. https://doi.org/10.1111/tbj.13944.
16. Yaghan R, Hamouri S, Ayoub NM, Yaghan L, Mazahreh T. A proposal of a clinically based classification for idiopathic granulomatous mastitis. Asian Pac J Cancer Prev. 2019;20:929–34. https://doi.org/10.31557/APJCP.2019.20.3.929.
17. Adams DH, Hubscher SG, Scott DG. Granulomatous mastitis—a rare cause of erythema nodosum. Postgrad Med J. 1987;63:581–2. https://doi.org/10.1136/pgmj.63.741.581.
18. Akın M, Karabacak H, Esendağlı G, Yavuz A, Gültekin S, Dikmen K, et al. Coexistence of idiopathic granulomatous mastitis and erythemanodosum: successful treatment with corticosteroids. Turk J Med Sci. 2017;47:1590–2. https://doi.org/10.3906/sag-1611-100.
19. Al-Khaffaf BH, Shanks JH, Bundred N. Erythema nodosum—an extramammary manifestation of granulomatous mastitis. Breast J. 2006;12:569–70. https://doi.org/10.1111/j.1524-4741.2006.00348.x.
20. Alungal J, Abdulla MC, Narayan R. Idiopathic granulomatous mastitis with erythema nodosum and polyarthritis. Reumatismo. 2016;68:97–9. https://doi.org/10.4081/reumatismo.2016.844.
21. Bes C, Soy M, Vardi S, Sengul N, Yilmaz F. Erythema nodosum associated with granulomatous mastitis: report of two cases. Rheumatol Int. 2010;30:1523–5. https://doi.org/10.1007/s00296-009-1109-y.
22. Binesh F, Shiryazdi M, Bagher Owlia M, Azimi S. Idiopathic granulomatous mastitis, erythema nodosum and bilateral ankle arthritis in an Iranian woman. BMJ Case Rep. 2013;2013:bcr2012007636. https://doi.org/10.1136/bcr-2012-007636.
23. Choi EC, Wong SBJ, Ho SJ. Idiopathic granulomatous mastitis and erythema nodosum—a unifying pathophysiology? Australas J Dermatol 2021. 2020;62:e149–53. https://doi.org/10.1111/ajd.13463.
24. Damade R, Pouchot J, Vinceneux P. Systemic manifestations of granulomatous mastitis. Presse Med. 1992;21:2155.
25. Fahmy J, Halabi-Tawil M, Bagot M, Tournant B, Petit A. Erythema nodosum during the course of idiopathic granulomatous mastitis. Ann Dermatol Venereol. 2015;142:46–9. https://doi.org/10.1016/j.annder.2014.09.009.
26. Fruchter R, Castilla C, Ng E, Pomeranz MK, Femia AN. Erythema nodosum in association with idiopathic granulomatous mastitis: a case series and review of the literature. J Eur Acad Dermatol Venereol. 2017;31:e391–3. https://doi.org/10.1111/jdv.14194.
27. Gumus M, Akkurt ZM, Gumus H. Is erythema nodosum coexisting with lesions of the breast a suggestive sign for idiopathic granulomatous mastitis? Turk J Surg. 2018;34:71–3. https://doi.org/10.5152/turkjsurg.2017.3161.
28. Jacquin-Porretaz C, Devalland C, Delapparent T, Nardin C, Dupond AS. Idiopathic granulomatous mastitis associated with erythema nodosum. Ann Dermatol Venereol. 2019;146:571–6. https://doi.org/10.1016/j.annder.2019.04.023.
29. Kageyama R, Ueda H, Hashizume H. A case of granulomatous mastitis, erythema nodosum and oligoarthralgia in a pregnant woman with high serum granulocyte-colony-stimulating factor. Eur J Dermatol. 2016;26:205–7. https://doi.org/10.1684/ejd.2015.2714.
30. Kalayci TO, Koruyucu MB, Apaydin M, Etit D, Varer M. Idiopathic granulomatous mastitis associated with erythema nodosum. Balkan Med J. 2016;33:228–31. https://doi.org/10.5152/balkanmedj.2015.150089.
31. Lucas R, Gussman D, Polis RL, Rattigan MI, Matulewicz TJ. Idiopathic granulomatous mastitis with erythema nodosum simulating breast abscess in pregnancy: a case report. Obstet Med. 2014;7:37–9. https://doi.org/10.1177/1753495X13502474.
32. Nakamura T, Yoshioka K, Miyashita T, Ikeda K, Ogawa Y, Inoue T, et al. Granulomatous mastitis complicated by arthralgia and erythema nodosum successfully treated with prednisolone and methotrexate. Intern Med. 2012;51:2957–60. https://doi.org/10.2169/internalmedicine.51.7846.

33. Nakamura Y, Yamaguchi M, Nakamura A, Muto M. Tender, red nodules and arthralgia in a young woman with mastitis. Clin Exp Dermatol. 2014;39:410–2. https://doi.org/10.1111/ced.12276.
34. Olfatbakhsh A, Beheshtian T, Djavid GE. Granulomatous mastitis, erythema nodosum, and oligoarthritis in a pregnant woman. Breast J. 2008;14:588–90. https://doi.org/10.1111/j.1524-4741.2008.00653.x.
35. Polat M, Kaya H. Plantar erythema nodosum associated with granulomatous mastitis. Indian J Dermatol Venereol Leprol. 2016;82:202–4. https://doi.org/10.4103/0378-6323.164219.
36. Salesi M, Karimifar M, Salimi F, Mahzouni P. A case of granulomatous mastitis with erythema nodosum and arthritis. Rheumatol Int. 2011;31:1093–5. https://doi.org/10.1007/s00296-009-1273-0.
37. Vural S, Ertop P, Ceyhan K, Şanli H. An unusual cause of oligoarthritis and erythema nodosum: idiopathic granulomatous mastitis. Arch Rheumatol. 2017;32:71–5. https://doi.org/10.5606/ArchRheumatol.2017.5952.
38. Weber JC, Gros D, Blaison G, Martin T, Storck D, Pasquali JL. Granulomatous mastitis, erythema nodosa and oligoarthritis. Apropos of a case. Rev Med Interne. 1994;15:190–2. https://doi.org/10.1016/s0248-8663(05)82147-2.
39. Zabetian S, Friedman BJ, McHargue C. A case of idiopathic granulomatous mastitis associated with erythema nodosum, arthritis, and reactive cough. JAAD Case Rep. 2016;2:125–7. https://doi.org/10.1016/j.jdcr.2016.01.011.
40. Irkorucu O. Granulomatous mastitis: a practical classification system. Isr Med Assoc J. 2016;18:307–8.
41. Irkorucu O. Granulomatous mastitis: we need a useful classification system. Am J Surg. 2018;216:642. https://doi.org/10.1016/j.amjsurg.2017.08.007.
42. Kaviani A, Vasigh M. Classification of the clinical presentation, severity, and response to treatment in idiopathic granulomatousis mastitis. Arch Breast Cancer [Internet]. 2021;8:1–3. https://doi.org/10.32768/abc.2021811-3.

Microbiology and Biological Markers

Natalie G. Johnson and Naim Kadoglou

1 Introduction

Idiopathic granulomatous mastitis (IGM) is a benign, inflammatory disease. It is a rare chronic condition of the breast. Wolloch and Kessler [1] described this disease of the breast in 1972 but the etiology is as yet unknown. The clinical presentation of IGM can mimic infection in over half of the cases reported. The differential of this presentation also includes breast cancer. IGM presents itself as an inflammation of the breast with recurrent relapses. It is reportedly more common in women of Asian, North African, or Hispanic heritage [2] and generally seen in women of reproductive age between 30 and 45 years who have had a pregnancy in the 5 years leading up to their presentation [3]. It has proven itself to be a diagnostic and therapeutic challenge and several modalities have been proposed in its management, including corticosteroids and surgery. The triggers and the exact pathophysiology of the disease as well as a gold standard of management are yet to be elucidated. This chapter aims to review the published theories, with regards to the microbiology, pathogenesis, pathways, and potential biomarker targets for management.

N. G. Johnson (✉)
The Royal Marsden Hospital, London, UK

N. Kadoglou
Imperial College, Breast Unit, London North West University Healthcare NHS Trust,
Northwick Park Hospital, Harrow, London, UK

© The Author(s), under exclusive license to Springer Nature Switzerland AG 2023 37
H. Koksal, N. Kadoglou (eds.), *Idiopathic Granulomatous Mastitis*,
https://doi.org/10.1007/978-3-031-30391-3_6

2 Pathophysiology and Pathogenesis

The exact triggers or causative agents for the disease are unknown, making it difficult to provide targeted therapy. The belief is that external factors or triggers disrupt the equilibrium that exists between the natural flora of the breast and the microenvironment resulting in a release of inflammatory factors and milk secretion that damages the epithelium of the breast. The overall theory suggests that epithelial damage leads to a local granulomatous inflammation. There is also the theory of an autoimmune pathophysiology that is supported by the positive response that patients display when treated with steroids and other immunosuppressant agents. The role of bacterial agents is often under discussion but not yet fully proven.

As noted, the current proposed pathophysiology of the disease, Fig. 1, starts with a trigger that causes the initial damage to the ductal epithelium in the breast. The luminal secretions then enters the surrounding lobular connective tissue. This inflammation that occurs locally leads to the infiltration of lymphocytes and macrophages to the affected area and ultimately the formation of a local granulomatous inflammatory response. This pathophysiological theory is supported by the

Fig. 1 Proposed pathogenesis of idiopathic granulomatous mastitis

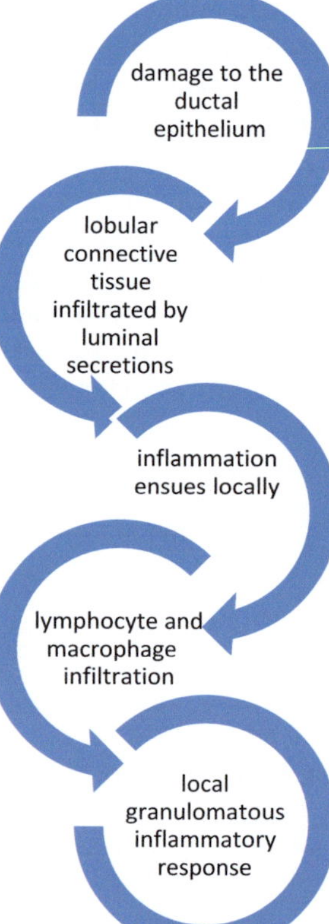

infiltration seen in histological specimens, the disease response to glucocorticoid treatment, and the identification of extra-mammarian manifestations of the disease [4].

3   Infection and IGM

With regards to infection, the most common bacteria associated with granulomas in breast abscesses is *Corynebacterium*. As it is part of the natural skin flora, there may be some overlap and confusion between colonization, infection, and contamination. Some authors have used the term cystic neutrophilic granulomatous mastitis to describe IGM associated with the isolation of this gram-positive bacillus [5].

Research published in 2003 by Taylor et al. identified *Corynebacterium* in more than half of their patients who were diagnosed histologically with granulomatous mastitis [6]. This study provided the initial association between *Corynebacterium* and IGM. The species most commonly identified in their research was *Corynebacterium kroppenstedtii*, which was noted in 14 of their 62 cases [5]. The presence of *Corynebacterium* has been confirmed by several subsequent studies granted with different rates of detection [6–8]. This may be accounted for by the inconsistencies of the detection techniques used in these reports as well as the differing test material sampled.

The nontuberculous bacteria, *Mycobacterium abscessus* and *Mycobacterium fortuitum*, have also been implicated in IGM [9]. These pathogens potentially respond to antituberculosis drugs triple therapy with a combination of linezolid, clarithromycin, tigecycline, and amikacin. Of the other bacteria thus far identified in cases of IGM, the most common pathogens include that of *Stenotrophomonas*, *Acinetobacter*, *Aspergillus*, *Pseudomonas*, *Brevundimonas*, and *Actinomyces* [10, 11].

In contrast, in another small retrospective study of 45 patients, the authors surmised that bacterial agents were unlikely involved in the etiology of IGM. They conducted molecular-based assays of flora including *Corynebacterium* spp. and other common infective agents. Their conclusion came following the lack of detection of bacterial DNA from their samples prior to intervention of any kind, whether surgical or steroid. There was a lack of evidence of any clinical benefit in those treated with antibiotics, as the treatment did not result in clinical recovery in the patients in the study [12].

4   Antibiotic Treatment in IGM

Antibiotic treatment proves beneficial in the case of complex IGM when there is superficial infection. Abscesses require the gold standard management of incision and drainage or aspiration as indicated. However, for superficial skin infections, there is no current consensus of treatment. In their paper published in 2019, Tan et al. noted resistance to penicillin of up to 70% of patients who tested positive for *Corynebacterium* with IGM [13]. Prior to this, Dobinson et al. [14] noted the resistance of *C. kroppenstedtii* to beta-lactam antibiotics. In this paper they recommended antibiotics such as doxycycline, clarithromycin, and rifampicin which are lipophilic in nature [14, 15].

5   Markers in Diagnosis and Investigations

5.1   *C-Reactive Protein and Interleukin-6*

Previous publications have noted the increase serum concentrations of interleukins (IL) in IGM. This included IL-8, IL-10, IL-17, IL-22, IL-23, and IL-33 [16–18]. A recent study by Huang et al. [19] confirmed this correlation with a particular difference noted in IL-6 levels in those with IGM. IL-6 is an endogenous pyrogen that induces the acute phase response [20]. IL-1 and TNF-alpha perform in the same manner. They noted significantly higher serum concentrations of IL-1 beta, tumor necrosis factor-alpha, IL-2, 6, 12p70, and 17A in IGM sufferers' vs control group without the disease. Of these, IL-6 proved to be significantly different in mild, moderate, and severe disease, sufferers having the highest levels. This study also showed a positive correlation between higher IL-6 levels and time to resolution. Factors such as skin ulceration, fistulae, bilateral disease, and high C-reactive protein (CRP) levels also correlated with longer time to resolution and risk of recurrence [19]. The above findings suggest CRP and IL-6 to be useful biomarkers for assessing disease severity in IGM.

5.2   *Neutrophil-to-Lymphocyte Ratio (NLR) and IGM*

The NLR is an inflammatory biomarker that has been recognized as a risk factor for recurrent disease and is associated with poor outcomes in cardiovascular diseases [21], solid cancers [22] such as hepatocellular carcinoma [23], and diseases such as Takayasu's arteritis [24]. Patients with recurrence of IGM were found to have a significantly higher preoperative NLR, which has been reported as an indicator of the severity of inflammation in autoimmune disease [24]. It is calculated by dividing absolute neutrophil count by absolute lymphocyte count. In the most recent Turkish paper, by Cetinkaya et al. [25], the preoperative NLR was found to predict recurrence. The sensitivity (62.5%) and specificity (84.8%) suggest it can be used to predict the recurrence of IGM and therefore would be a useful tool in the follow-up setting as a predictive tool [25]. In this particular study, CRP was not measured but it is understood to be essential in the assessment of inflammation alongside NLR.

5.3 sTREM-1 (Soluble Triggering Receptor Expressed on Myeloid Cells) and IGM

In a Turkish case-controlled study published earlier this year, with 60 patients that were further subcategorized as active or in remission, high sTREM-1 levels were found to contribute to the inflammation seen in IGM. The innate immune cells, which function by identifying and eliminating pathogens that lead to infection, include natural killer cells, neutrophils, basophils, dendritic cells, macrophages, mast cells, and eosinophils. TREM-1 is expressed by these cells and plays a role in the process of inflammation. Apart from its increased effect on the expression of cell activation markers on the cell surface, it stimulates chemokine and cytokine release as well as the inflammatory responses mediated by neutrophils and monocytes [26].

Gao et al. [27] reported that the production of many cytokines increased with the activation of TREM-1, making it a suitable target, particularly in the therapy-resistant group of patients. They included monocyte chemoattractant protein-1 and protein-3, interleukin-6 and interleukin-8, tumor necrosis alpha, and macrophage-stimulating protein 1-alpha also.

5.4 Interleukin-33 in IGM

IL-33 belongs to the IL-1 cytokine family and serves to regulate transcription as an intracellular nuclear factor. It also activates the sST2 (suppression of tumorigenicity receptor complex), which is upstream of T-helper type 2 immune and associated inflammatory responses. sST2 serves to downregulate the function of IL-33 and also has anti-inflammatory properties that are activated by IL-33 [18, 28, 29].

In a study by Yigitbasi et al. [18], it was shown that IL-33 levels were markedly higher in IGM patients compared to patients diagnosed with breast cancer, whereas ST2 levels were markedly lower in the IGM group vs the breast cancer group. However, the levels of IL-33 were seen to be elevated in both groups when compared to the control group. With these findings, they concluded that IL-33 and ST2 levels in conjunction with radiological and histological findings could help to distinguish between IGM and breast cancer [18].

Serum prolactin is useful to exclude hyperprolactinemia and serum angiotensin-converting enzyme is useful in those patients with extra-mammarian signs suggestive of systemic inflammatory diseases.

The erythrocyte sedimentation rate (ESR) and CRP are elevated in IGM as in breast abscesses but less so in breast cancer. In order to rule out infectious etiology, tests for bacteria, mycobacteria, and fungi should also be undertaken. With systemic inflammatory disease amongst the differentials, literature has suggested the use of tests for ANA and dsDNA as part of the investigations; however, the results have not been shown to be statistically significant when compared to the control group [4, 30, 31].

As discussed in the pathophysiology and pathogenesis, serum biomarkers in patients with IGM are proving to be useful in the prediction of severity and recurrence and should be considered in the diagnostic workup as indicated, in particular IL-6 and CRP as biomarkers for disease severity and NLR as a predictor of recurrence. IL-33 has been proposed as a biomarker to distinguish between breast cancer and IGM alongside radiological and histological diagnostic findings.

6 Summary

The disease process of idiopathic granulomatous mastitis is believed to be a result of initial ductal epithelial damage. The gold standard of treatment and the duration of intervention are not yet standardized with steroids, antibiotics, methotrexate, and surgery as being the most commonly used interventions. *Corynebacterium*, particularly *Corynebacterium kroppenstedtii*, is the bacterial agent mostly identified as a causative agent in the majority of cases reported. It has been seen as resistant to beta-lactam antibiotics but responsive to antibiotics such as doxycycline, rifampicin, and clarithromycin.

Serum CRP and IL-6 levels and NLR are proposed biomarkers for the measurement of disease severity and time to resolution in patients with IGM. TREM-1 and IL33 are triggers that have been implicated in the pathway of the disease process and present themselves as potential targets in the management of IGM. The majority of literature presented is retrospective as the disease is rare, making the elucidation of management modalities challenging. Indeed, further research is required and recent publications prove promising in the guidance of management to date.

References

1. Kessler E, Wolloch Y. Granulomatous mastitis: a lesion clinically simulating carcinoma. Am J Clin Pathol. 1972;58:642–6. https://doi.org/10.1093/ajcp/58.6.642.
2. Martinez-Ramos D, Simon-Monterde L, Suelves-Piqueres C, Queralt-Martin R, Granel-Villach L, Laguna-Sastre JM, et al. Idiopathic granulomatous mastitis: a systematic review of 3060 patients. Breast J. 2019;25:1245–50. https://doi.org/10.1111/tbj.13446.
3. Altintoprak F, Kivilcim T, Ozkan OV. Aetiology of idiopathic granulomatous mastitis. World J Clin Cases. 2014;2:852–8. https://doi.org/10.12998/wjcc.v2.i12.852.
4. Sheybani F, Naderi HR, Gharib M, Sarvghad M, Mirfeizi Z. Idiopathic granulomatous mastitis: long-discussed but yet-to-be-known. Autoimmunity. 2016;49:236–9. https://doi.org/1 0.3109/08916934.2016.1138221.
5. Taylor GB, Paviour SD, Musaad S, Jones WO, Holland DJ. A clinicopathological review of 34 cases of inflammatory breast disease showing an association between corynebacteria infection and granulomatous mastitis. Pathology. 2003;35:109–19.
6. Kutsuna S, Mezaki K, Nagamatsu M, Kunimatsu J, Yamamoto K, Fujiya Y, et al. Two cases of granulomatous mastitis caused by Corynebacterium kroppenstedtii infection in nulliparous

young women with hyperprolactinemia. Intern Med. 2015;54:1815–8. https://doi.org/10.2169/internalmedicine.54.4254.

7. Bercot B, Kannengiesser C, Oudin C, Grandchamp B, Sanson-le Pors MJ, Mouly S, et al. First description of NOD2 variant associated with defective neutrophil responses in a woman with granulomatous mastitis related to corynebacteria. J Clin Microbiol. 2009;47:3034–7. https://doi.org/10.1128/JCM.00561-09.

8. Mathelin C, Riegel P, Chenard MP, Tomasetto C, Brettes JP. Granulomatous mastitis and corynebacteria: clinical and pathologic correlations. Breast J. 2005;11:357. https://doi.org/10.1111/j.1075-122X.2005.21562.x.

9. Sanchez Eluchans N, Barberis C, Cittadini R, Ozuna Villca AM, Veiga MF, Vilches V, et al. Corynebacterium kroppenstedtii breast infections: report of four cases. Rev Argent Microbiol. 2021;53:304–8. https://doi.org/10.1016/j.ram.2021.01.002.

10. Li XQ, Wu HL, Yuan JP, et al. Bacteria associated with granulomatous lobular mastitis and the potential for personalized therapy. J Investig Surg. 2022;35:164–70. https://doi.org/10.1080/08941939.2020.1833262.

11. Wang J, Xu H, Li Z, Li F, Yang Y, Yu X, et al. Pathogens in patients with granulomatous lobular mastitis. Int J Infect Dis. 2019;81:123–7. https://doi.org/10.1016/j.ijid.2019.01.034.

12. Kivilcim T, Altintoprak F, Memis B, Ferhatoğlu MF, Kartal A, Dikicier E, et al. Role of bacteriological agents in idiopathic granulomatous mastitis: real or not? Eur J Breast Health. 2018;15:32–6. https://doi.org/10.5152/ejbh.2018.4249.

13. Tan QT, Tay SP, Gudi MA, Nadkarni NV, Lim SH, Chuwa EWL. Granulomatous mastitis and factors associated with recurrence: an 11-year single-Centre study of 113 patients in Singapore. World J Surg. 2019;43:1737–45. https://doi.org/10.1007/s00268-019-05014-x.

14. Dobinson HC, Anderson TP, Chambers ST, Doogue MP, Seaward L, Werno AM. Antimicrobial treatment options for granulomatous mastitis caused by Corynebacterium species. J Clin Microbiol. 2015;53:2895–9. https://doi.org/10.1128/JCM.00760-15.

15. Paviour S, Musaad S, Roberts S, Taylor G, Taylor S, Shore K, et al. Corynebacterium species isolated from patients with mastitis. Clin Infect Dis. 2002;35:1434–40. https://doi.org/10.1086/344463.

16. Koksal H, Vatansev H, Artac H, Kadoglou N. The clinical value of interleukins-8, −10, and −17 in idiopathic granulomatous mastitis. Clin Rheumatol. 2020;39:1671–7. https://doi.org/10.1007/s10067-020-04925-8.

17. Saydam M, Yilmaz KB, Sahin M, Yanik H, Akinci M, Yilmaz I, et al. New findings on autoimmune etiology of idiopathic granulomatous mastitis: serum IL-17, IL-22 and IL-23 levels of patients. J Investig Surg. 2021;34:993–7. https://doi.org/10.1080/08941939.2020.1725190.

18. Yigitbasi MR, Guntas G, Atak T, Sonmez C, Yalman H, Uzun H. The role of interleukin-33 as an inflammatory marker in differential diagnosis of idiopathic granulomatous mastitis and breast cancer. J Investig Surg. 2017;30:272–6. https://doi.org/10.1080/08941939.2016.1240270.

19. Huang YM, Lo C, Cheng CF, Lu CH, Hsieh SC, Li KJ. Serum C-reactive protein and interleukin-6 levels as biomarkers for disease severity and clinical outcomes in patients with idiopathic granulomatous mastitis. J Clin Med. 2021;10:2077. https://doi.org/10.3390/jcm10102077.

20. Kany S, Vollrath JT, Relja B. Cytokines in inflammatory disease. Int J Mol Sci. 2019;20:6008. https://doi.org/10.3390/ijms20236008.

21. Kim S, Eliot M, Koestler DC, Wu WC, Kelsey KT. Association of neutrophil-to-lymphocyte ratio with mortality and cardiovascular disease in the Jackson heart study and modification by the Duffy antigen variant. JAMA Cardiol. 2018;3:455–62. https://doi.org/10.1001/jamacardio.2018.1042.

22. Templeton AJ, McNamara MG, Šeruga B, Vera-Badillo FE, Aneja P, Ocaña A, et al. Prognostic role of neutrophil-to-lymphocyte ratio in solid tumors: a systematic review and meta-analysis. J Natl Cancer Inst. 2014;106:dju124. https://doi.org/10.1093/jnci/dju124.

23. Zheng J, Cai J, Li H, Zeng K, He L, Fu H, et al. Neutrophil to lymphocyte ratio and platelet to lymphocyte ratio as prognostic predictors for hepatocellular carcinoma patients with various

treatments: a meta-analysis and systematic review. Cell Physiol Biochem. 2017;44:967–81. https://doi.org/10.1159/000485396.

24. Pan L, Du J, Li T, Liao H. Platelet-to-lymphocyte ratio and neutrophil-to-lymphocyte ratio associated with disease activity in patients with Takayasu's arteritis: a case-control study. BMJ Open. 2017;7:e014451. https://doi.org/10.1136/bmjopen-2016-014451.

25. Cetinkaya OA, Celik SU, Terzioglu SG, Eroglu A. The predictive value of the neutrophil-to-lymphocyte and platelet-to-lymphocyte ratio in patients with recurrent idiopathic granulomatous mastitis. Eur J Breast Health. 2020;16:61–5. https://doi.org/10.5152/ejbh.2019.5187.

26. Ates D, Doner HC, Kurban S, Koksal H. The effect of soluble TREM-1 in idiopathic granulomatous mastitis. Immunol Investig. 2022;51:839–50. https://doi.org/10.1080/08820139.2021.1879846.

27. Gao S, Yi Y, Xia G, Yu C, Ye C, Tu F, et al. The characteristics and pivotal roles of triggering receptor expressed on myeloid cells-1 in autoimmune diseases. Autoimmun Rev. 2019;18:25–35. https://doi.org/10.1016/j.autrev.2018.07.008.

28. De la Fuente M, MacDonald TT, Hermoso MA. The IL-33/ST2 axis: role in health and disease. Cytokine Growth Factor Rev. 2015;26:615–23. https://doi.org/10.1016/j.cytogfr.2015.07.017.

29. Shang J, Zhao J, Wu X, Xu Y, Xie J, Zhao J. Interleukin-33 promotes inflammatory cytokine production in chronic airway inflammation. Biochem Cell Biol. 2015;93:359–66. https://doi.org/10.1139/bcb-2014-0163.

30. Altintoprak F, Karakece E, Kivilcim T, Dikicier E, Cakmak G, Celebi F, et al. Idiopathic granulomatous mastitis: an autoimmune disease? ScientificWorldJournal. 2013;2013:148727. https://doi.org/10.1155/2013/148727.

31. Koksal H. The clinical utility of autoantibodies in patients with idiopathic granulomatous mastitis. J Investig Surg. 2022;35:325–9. https://doi.org/10.1080/08941939.2020.1861666.

Imaging Studies in Idiopathic Granulomatous Mastitis

Nevin Sekmenli

1   Mammography

Idiopathic granulomatous mastitis (IGM), a chronic, benign, and inflammatory disease of the breast, is frequently confused with malignant lesions due to its clinical and radiological findings. The first radiological step in the breast imaging algorithm is mammography. The sensitivity of mammography is lower among the young population due to the dense breast pattern [1–3].

Mammographic findings are reported as negative in 50% of cases in the literature. However, in some cases, mammographic findings are suspicious enough to easily suggest malignancy [3]. The mammographic images may vary from one case to another. Regarding mammography, an asymmetric density with no parenchymal distortion or microcalcifications and/or a mass with benign or suspicious properties and focal asymmetric density may be seen. The most common mammographic appearance in IGM is asymmetric density. In previous studies, dense or heterogeneous dense breast patterns were observed in more than half of the cases [4]. In a study by Fazzio et al. [5], a moderate-sized focal asymmetry demonstrating the region of palpable mass was observed as the most widespread finding on the mammography [5].

Focal asymmetry (Fig. 1), asymmetric fibroglandular increase in density (Fig. 2), structural distortion (Fig. 3), nipple retraction (Fig. 4), retroareolar asymmetric density (Fig. 5), trabecular thickening (Fig. 6), irregular or ellipsoid-shape density (Fig. 7), and multifocal involvement can be detected in the non-dense breasts. Additionally, there may be a thickening of the skin in the superficially involved areas.

N. Sekmenli (✉)
Department of Radiology, Saglik Bilimleri University, Hamidiye Faculty of Medicine, Ministry of Health Konya City Hospital, Konya, Türkiye

H. Koksal, N. Kadoglou (eds.), *Idiopathic Granulomatous Mastitis*,
https://doi.org/10.1007/978-3-031-30391-3_7

Fig. 1 Mediolateral oblique mammograms of the right and left breasts of a 41-year-old woman with IGM. A focal asymmetric density is seen in the upper portion of the right breast (arrow)

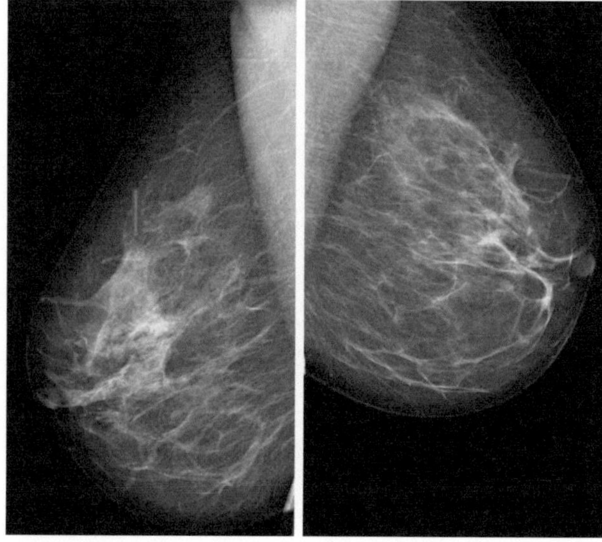

Fig. 2 A 36-year-old woman with IGM. Bilateral mediolateral oblique mammogram demonstrates regional asymmetry with indistinct margins in the middle upper portion of the left breast. The left breast size has increased globally

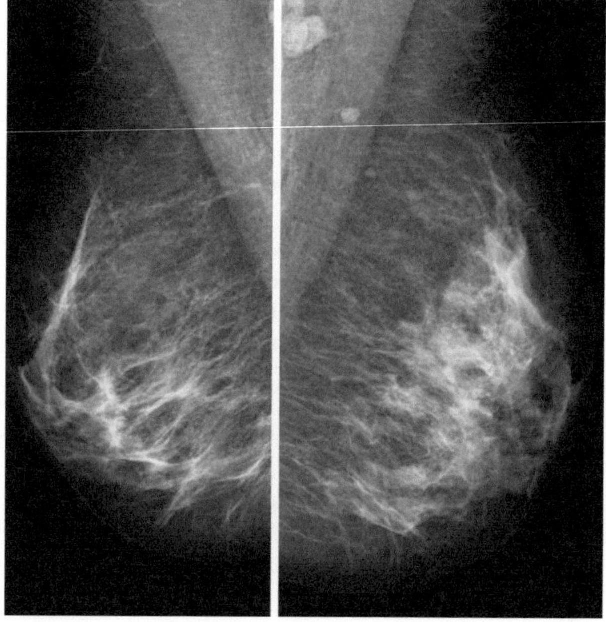

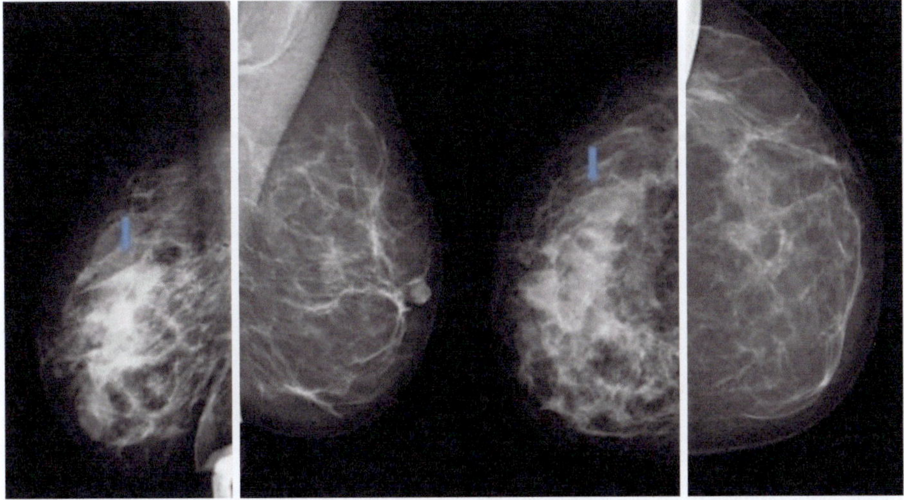

Fig. 3 Bilateral mediolateral oblique and craniocaudal mammograms of a 38-year-old woman with IGM. A focal asymmetric density with indistinct margins is seen in the upper outer quadrant of the right breast (arrows)

Fig. 4 Bilateral mediolateral oblique mammography of a patient with pathologically proven diagnosis of IGM. Skin thickening and nipple retraction of the left breast is seen (arrow). Regional asymmetry in the retroareolar and lower region of the left breast is noticed. A well-circumscribed solitary mass in the upper right breast has simple cystic features sonographically

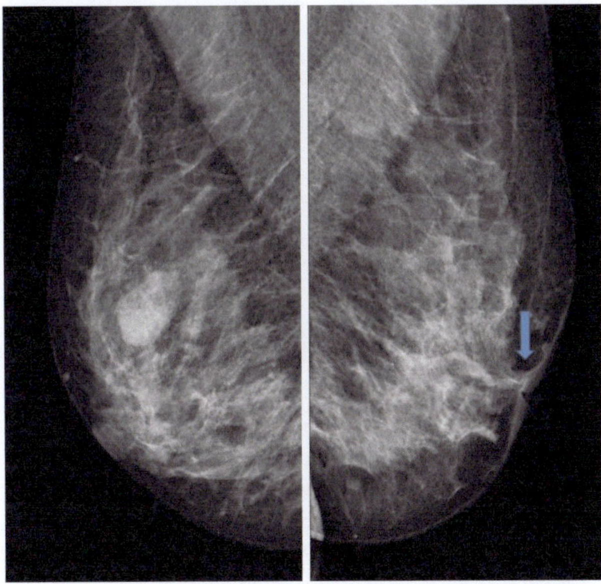

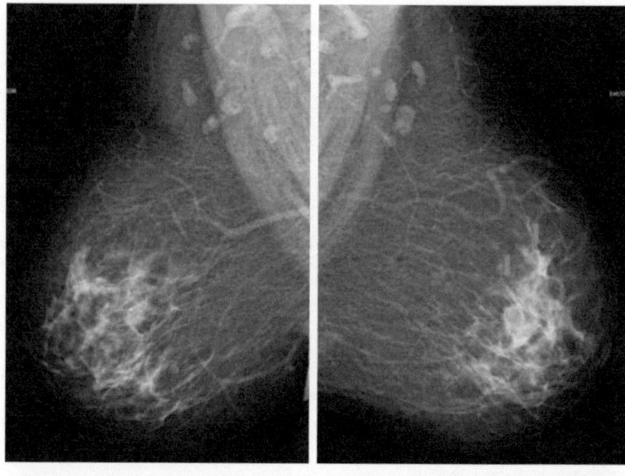

Fig. 5 Bilateral mediolateral oblique mammogram of a 28-year-old woman with IGM on the left breast. There is a regional asymmetry and slightly parenchymal distortion in the retroareolar region of the left breast (arrows)

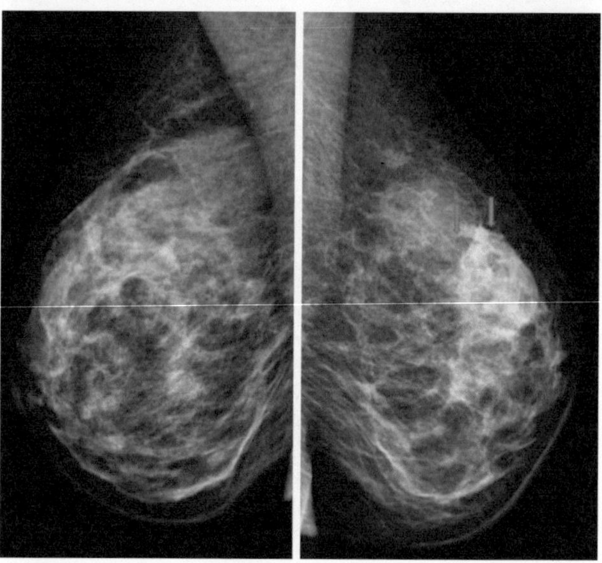

Fig. 6 IGM on the left breast in a woman. She has a palpable mass in the upper outer quadrant of the left breast. Bilateral mediolateral oblique mammogram demonstrates a large mass-like density with trabecular thickening in the upper quadrant of the left breast (arrows)

The cases of inflammatory breast cancer (IBC) present with similar manifestations. However, IBC characteristically involves over one-third of the breast skin, whereas IGM seldom involves the skin extensively [6].

In many patients, the affected breast is slightly larger than the opposite breast, especially in a mediolateral oblique (MLO) view (Fig. 2) [5].

IGM lesions can be observed in each quadrant of the breasts without any association with a specific quadrant.

In general, there is no relationship between IGM and calcifications [5, 7]. Fazzio et al. [5] reported that calcifications are a very rare mammographic finding of granulomatous mastitis via a single case appearing as segmental coarse heterogeneous calcifications [5].

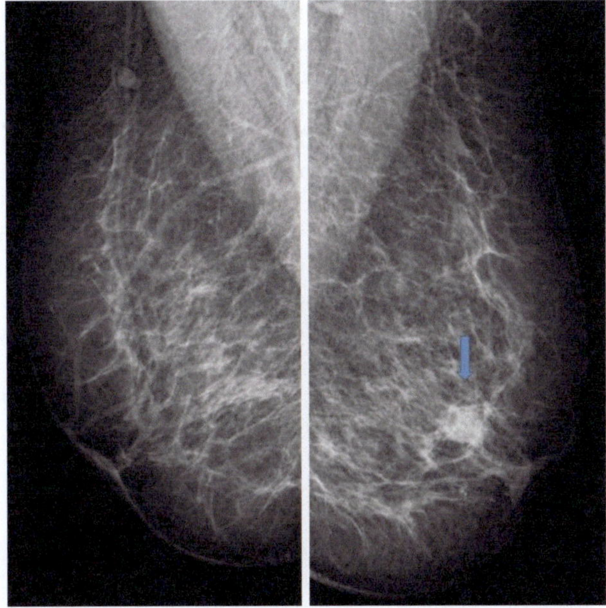

Fig. 7 Bilateral mediolateral oblique mammogram of a 28-year-old woman with IGM on the left breast. A nodular density with indistinct margins is seen in the retroareolar region of the left breast (arrow). Fibroglandular texture distribution is symmetrical in both breasts

2 Ultrasonography

Since IGM is encountered more commonly among premenopausal women presenting with mastitis and mass-like findings, the first-line diagnostic tool is examination through breast ultrasonography (US), rather than mammography and breast magnetic resonance imaging (MRI). Ultrasonography is a very valuable modality in IGM in the posttreatment follow-up phase, as well as its contribution to determining the diagnosis. While the sensitivity of US in detecting lesions is high, its specificity is low in the differential diagnosis of the lesions.

In addition to the algorithm for identified findings, the radiologist's comments and recommendations should also be recorded in the breast imaging report. Therefore, the use of the Breast Imaging Reporting and Data System (BI-RADS) classification has been created and, thus, has enabled such interpretations to be noted in standardized form [8]. The score of BI-RADS US includes the definition of the lesion seen, the degree of suspicion, which lesions should be biopsied, and recommendations to the clinician. BI-RADS 2 refers to benign lesions with no risk of malignancy.

In a previous study, 90% and 10% of IGM patients were reported to be defined as BI-RADS 3 and BI-RADS 4 categories sonographically, respectively [3]. IGM often mimics breast cancer clinically and radiologically, and the cases are commonly diagnosed as breast cancer initially [9]. Since the risk of breast cancer does not increase because of IGM diagnosis throughout the lifetime, the correct diagnosis is important to avoid unnecessary mastectomy. Therefore, US investigation is greatly beneficial in the differential diagnosis.

The most common sonographic finding in IGM is usually in the form of interconnected hypoechoic masses with irregular, ill-defined, and angled contours, including sinus tracts extending into the neighboring parenchyma in heterogeneous echoes in the peripheral sections of the breast (Figs. 8 and 9) [2, 5]. The lesions are almost always seen as parallel-orientated in the parenchyma.

Other common sonographic findings include features such as thickening of the breast skin (Fig. 10), enlargement of the ductal structures (Fig. 11), mass-like parenchymal distortion (Fig. 12), uniform or heterogeneous masses with regular contours (Fig. 13), global edema in the breast tissue (Fig. 14), parenchymal heterogeneity (Fig. 15), accumulated dense abscess-like contents (Fig. 16), tract formations opening to the skin or extending to the subcutaneous parenchyma (Fig. 15), and hypoechogenic areas casting a focal acoustic shadow (Fig. 17). Irregular contours, microlobulated angulations, and heterogeneous parenchymal areas often raise the suspicion of malignancy (Fig. 18).

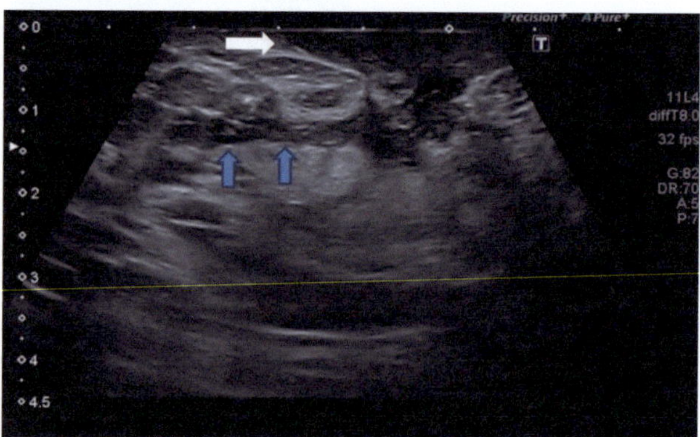

Fig. 8 Idiopathic granulomatous mastitis: a 30-year-old woman. Tubular connection (arrows up) extending between the breast lobules and subcutaneous tissue. Subcutaneous collection is seen (arrow to right)

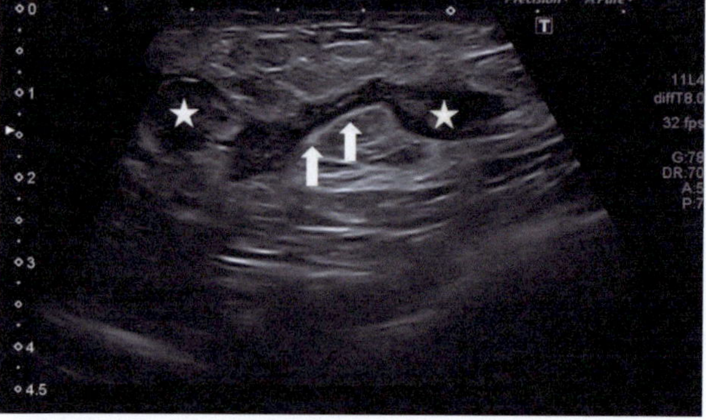

Fig. 9 A 36-year-old woman with IGM. Hypoechoic nodular structures (stars) and tubular connection (arrows)

Fig. 10 A 36-year-old woman with IGM. Multiple irregular hypoechoic masses and collections with tubular connection with fingerlike aspects and thickening of the skin (arrows)

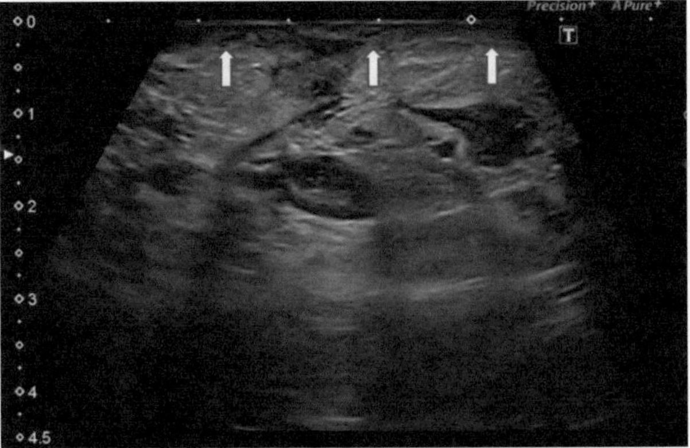

Fig. 11 A 32-year-old woman with IGM. Hypoechoic nodular structure (star) with ductal ectasia (arrows)

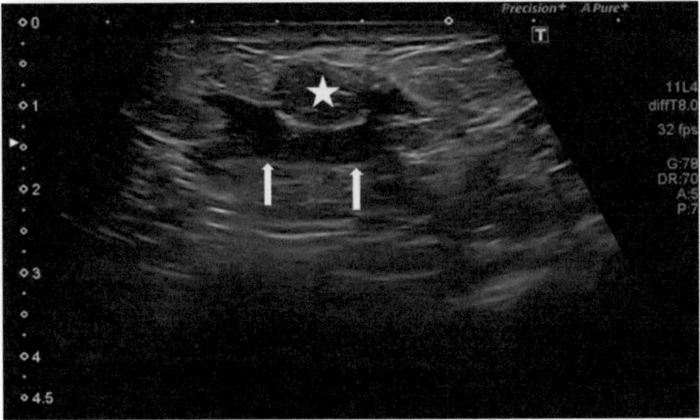

Fig. 12 Idiopathic granulomatous mastitis: a 30-year-old woman. Ill-defined hypoechoic concentrated collection (arrows) is connected with nodular hypoechoic structure (star)

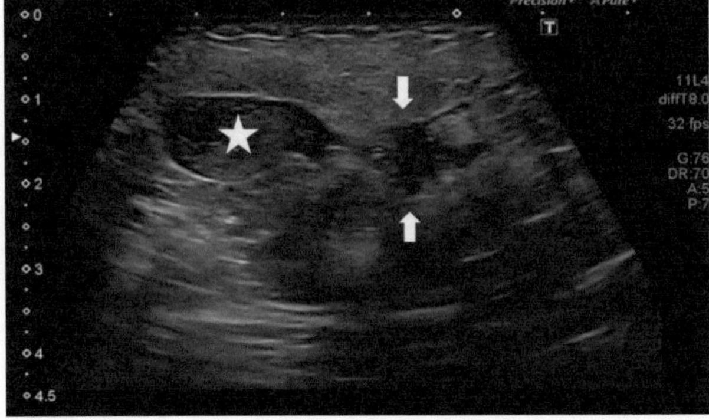

Fig. 13 A 36-year-old woman with IGM. She presented with a palpable mass. Ultrasound showed well-defined ovoid-shaped hypoechoic mass with posterior acoustic shadow

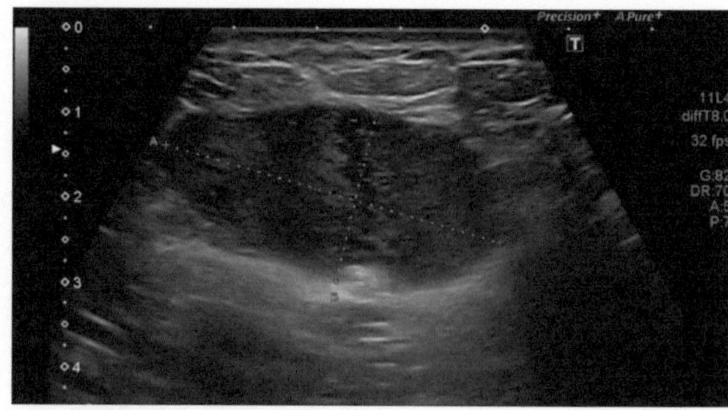

Fig. 14 A 29-year-old woman with IGM. Global edema in the breast tissue with focal sonolucent collection

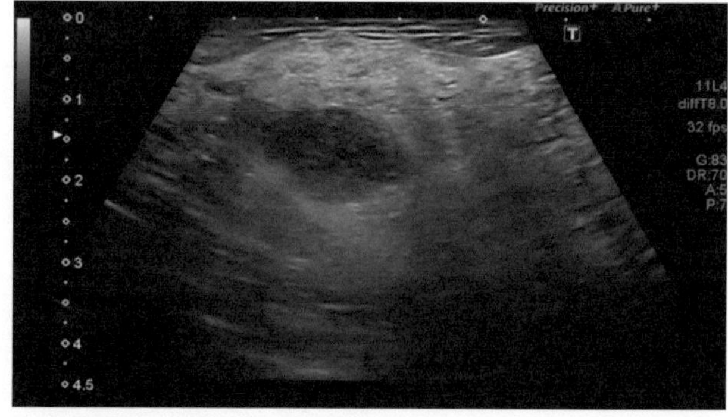

Fig. 15 A 32-year-old woman with IGM. Increased subcutaneous collection (arrows) with parenchymal edema and hypoechoic collections with tubular connection with fingerlike aspects

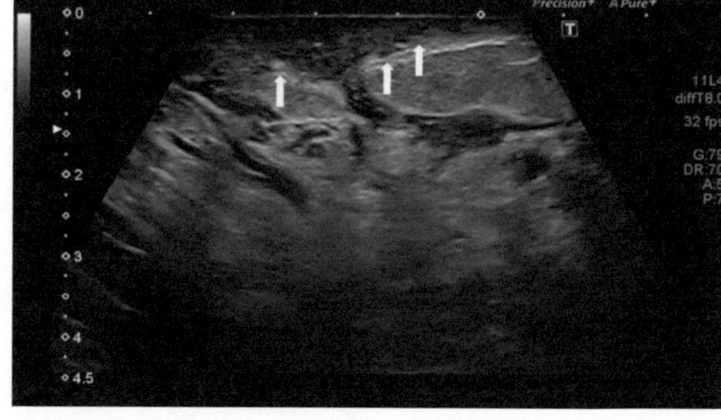

Fig. 16 A 30-year-old woman with IGM. A well-defined, abscess-like hypoechoic fluid-filled lesion

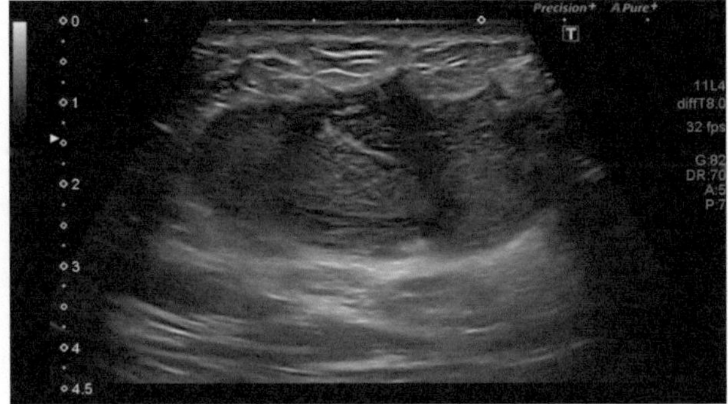

Fig. 17 Idiopathic granulomatous mastitis: a 26-year-old woman. Hypoechoic collection with fingerlike aspects and posterior acoustic shadows (curved arrows)

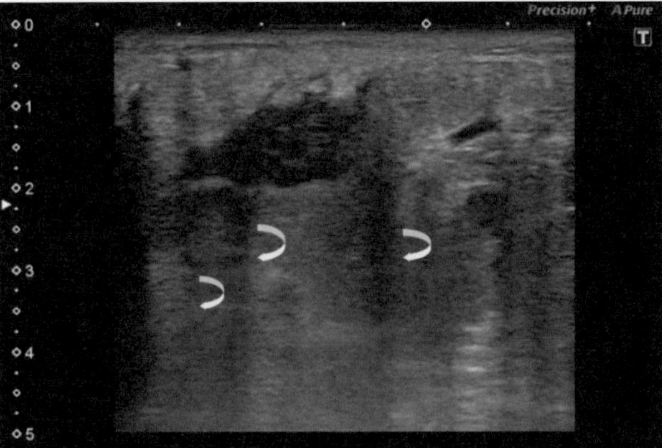

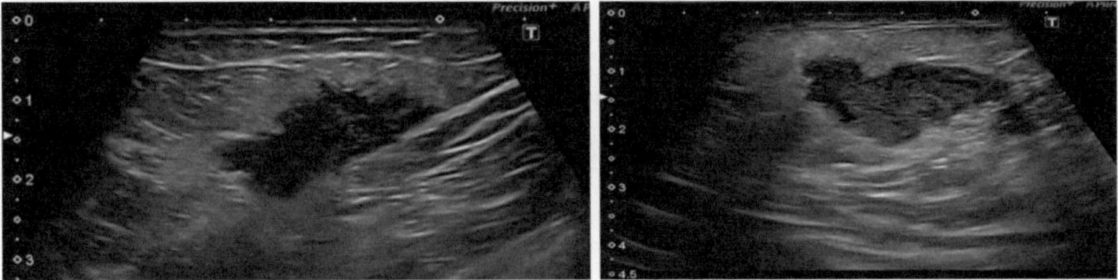

Fig. 18 A 36-year-old woman with IGM. Hypoechoic masses with irregular, microlobulated contours in the same breast and peripheral parenchymal edema

Long-term multiple fluid collections and abscess cavities are detected in advanced cases (Figs. 10 and 19). At this stage, fistulae are often observed on the skin (Fig. 20). In a study carried out by Teke et al. [10], it was stated that while the formation of abscesses and fistulae with echogenic debris encompassed by hyperechoic margins and posterior enhancement were detected in 27.08% of the patients, 14.58% of patients had focal hypoechoic parenchymal heterogeneity with indistinct border [10].

In a study in which Toprak and Gunduz [11] compared IGM with other types of mastitis (OM) in 95 patients based on US findings, it was reported that while palpable masses, fistulae, mass-like lesions with irregular margins accompanying tubular connections, and abscesses were more common in patients with IGM, ductal ectasia and periductal thickening were more widespread in those with OM. In the same study, the researchers also stated that albeit its higher incidence among OM patients, calcification was rarely observed in either group [11].

US investigation also provides a specific advantage in therapeutic or diagnostic aspiration in patients with abscesses and dense fluid collection.

In patients with axillary lymphadenopathy, US also helps to differentiate between the benign-malignant lymph nodes by determining the hilar echo and morphology of the lymph node along with its cortex thickness and shape (Fig. 21).

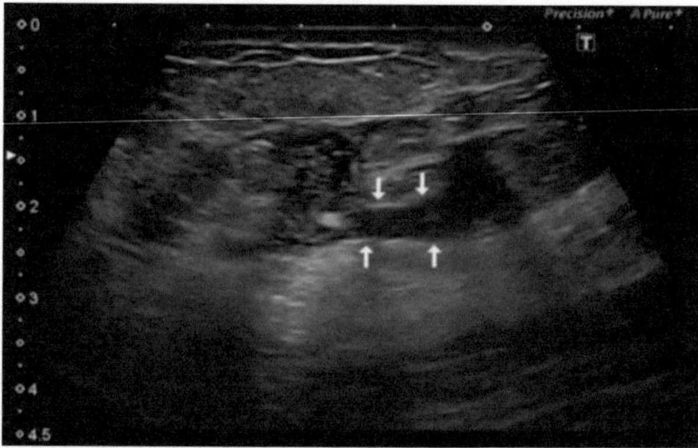

Fig. 19 A 32 -year-old woman with IGM. Hypoechoic masses with irregular, microlobulated contours with tubular connection (arrows)

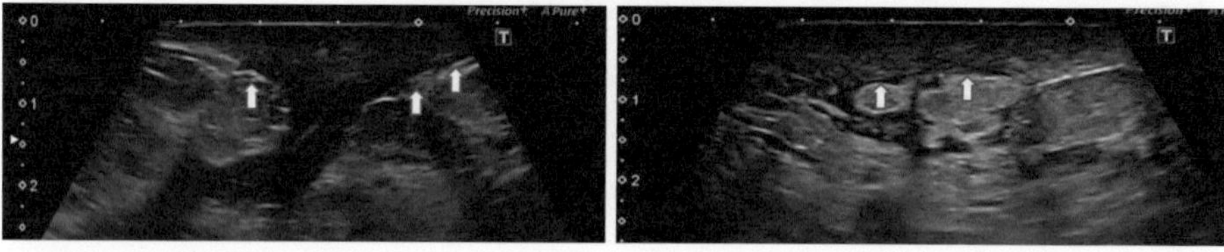

Fig. 20 A 29 -year-old woman with IGM. There are two pictures: subcutaneous wide collections (arrows) with abscess in the same patient

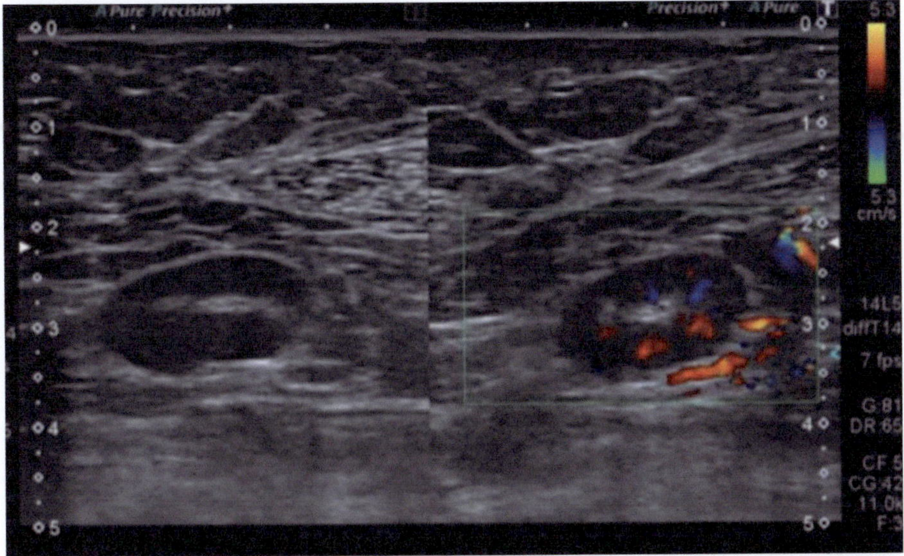

Fig. 21 An axillary reactive lymph node in an IGM patient. Central regular vascularity distribution is seen in color Doppler imaging with symmetrical cortical thickness

2.1 Doppler Ultrasonography

Doppler ultrasonography (US) permits the visualization of flow direction and velocity within a user-defined area. It is also another beneficial tool in guiding biopsies. On Doppler US, an arterial and venous vascularity increase is observed in the solid components of the lesion and the surrounding parenchyma with increased inflammation in IGM cases (Fig. 22). Spectral analysis findings in IGM are not specific [1].

Thus, selecting a safe area away from vascular structures where the biopsy needle will trace is to be achieved. However, if granulomatous mastitis is still suspected, the tissue sample should be obtained from the more vascular parts of the lesion in order to yield an accurate histological diagnosis [12, 13].

Fistulization of the skin, foci of abscesses, and skin changes are incredibly beneficial in the differential diagnosis of IGM. However, in the presence of mass-like lesions with unclear contours and where there are no inflammatory findings, it is very difficult to distinguish benign-malignant lesions using B-mode US examination alone, and so in such a situation, the diagnostic efficiency of sonoelastography is utilized.

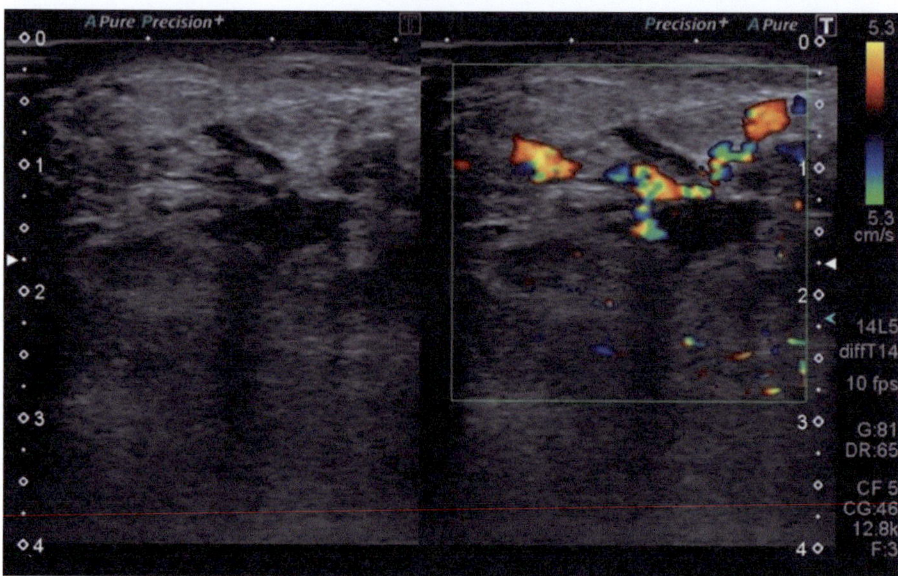

Fig. 22 A 37-year-old woman with IGM. A hypoechoic mass with irregular, microlobulated contours which has increased flow in color Doppler

2.2 Sonoelastography

Elastography is a significant investigation method developed in recent years as a special technique of conventional US allowing tissue elasticity to be measured. Undoubtedly, the most significant contribution of elastography to routine clinical practice is to reduce the number of unnecessary biopsies and follow-ups and to prevent false-negative findings by differentiating between BI-RADS 3 and 4A lesions. The elastographic investigation based on the evaluation of tissue stiffness is a less subjective, more sensitive, specific, and repeatable modality in distinguishing between benign and malignant lesions [14]. There are two different methods of elastographic investigation: shear-wave elastography (SWE) and compression elastography, also known as strain elastography (SE). SE is the general term of the method measuring the displacement of tissues by using the internal or external mild compression stimuli. SE is also a method based on the principle that the displacement in the tissue to which it is returned to its previous position after the compression is ended. The displacement of the tissue is calculated on the longitudinal plane where compression is performed. As the tissue stiffness increases, the response to displacement due to the compression decreases. The strain levels of normal breast tissue, adipose tissue, ductal carcinoma in situ, and infiltrative breast carcinoma are different. The displacement develops more easily in soft tissues such as fat, and both the displacement and returning of the lesion to its former position occur slowly in malignant processes and solid lesions due to fibrosis. Compared to all other breast tissue and lesions, infiltrative ductal carcinoma is the hardest tissue [15]. In coding to show solid lesions in color, while blue generally represents the hardest tissues, green and red represent the moderately solid and soft tissues, respectively. However, it should be kept in mind that there may be differences between the color preferences and software in terms of the settings of different devices.

In the characterization of benign vs malignant breast lesions, various scoring systems and parameters based on the SE method have been used. The most frequently used systems are the Tsukuba scoring, the E/B-mode ratio (measured by dividing the length of a lesion on elastography to the length of the lesion on B-mode US), and the strain ratio, which is calculated by the ratio of mean lesion strain to surrounding fatty tissue at the same depth [16].

Also called the 5-point color (5P) scoring, the Tsukuba scoring system is based on the evaluation of the lesion under the surrounding tissue in colored maps created with three main colors (solid tissues in blue, soft tissues in red, and moderately hard tissues in green) [17]. If equally hard or softer than the surrounding tissue, the lesion is called score 1; if the soft and hard components are together, the lesion is classified as score 2; if the lesion is hard when compared to the surrounding tissue but smaller in size than the B-mode, it is scored as 3; if hard compared to the surrounding tissue and the same as the B-mode, the lesion is classified as score 4, and if it looks hard regarding the surrounding tissue but larger than the B-mode in size, the lesion is classified as score 5 [18]. The lesions with scores 1 to 3 are likely to be benign, while those with scores 4 and 5 are considered to be suspicious. In a meta-analysis investigating 22 SE studies where the Tsukuba scoring system was mostly used, the average sensitivity and specificity rates were found to be 83% and 84% in distinguishing between benign and malignant lesions, respectively [19].

In the E/B system obtained from the dimensional values of the lesion, the measurements are achieved by dividing the measurement received from the elastography using the transverse length of the lesion by the measurement from the B-mode image. While the malignant lesions seem to be larger than the B-mode, due to the loss of elasticity caused by the stromal and desmoplastic reactions in the lesion area and surrounding tissue, the benign lesions appear to be smaller on elastography [20]. If the E/B ratio is less than 1, it is in favor of a benign lesion (sensitivity 100%, specificity 95%) [21].

The third method in the evaluation of SE is the strain index (SI). Concerning adipose tissue, the ratio obtained by placing the regions of interest (ROI) first to the lesion and then to the subcutaneous adipose tissue is a semiquantitative value [22]. In previous studies, SI has been found to increase in malignant lesions. Based on the literature, while specificity for the strain ratio were stated to range from 83% to 87%, sensitivity was reported to be between 88% and 94% [23–25].

In SE, the severity of external compression is a practitioner-dependent procedure, and different strain index values can be determined in the same tissue varying from one practitioner to another. Such a challenge also results in the analysis to be user-dependent and the findings to be subjective [26].

SWE is an elastography method measuring tissue elasticity without the need for external compression. The impulsive pulse generated by the US device induces both the displacement of the adjacent tissues and the formation of shear waves radiating in the transverse plane, perpendicular to the applied pulse [26]. The wave velocity formed by US is proportional to the hardness of the tissue, and the hardness of the lesion is in the form of objective numerical data that can be measured by the velocity of the wave obtained from the tissue. The optimum image is obtained from lesions up to 4 cm to the skin surface, and satisfactory figures may not be obtained from deeper tissues and lesions. The important advantage of SWE, unlike SE, is that its intra- and inter-practitioner variability is more consistent [27]. Shear-wave velocity (SWV) as a unit of elasticity is measured in terms of m/sec or as the kilopascal (kPa) of Young's modulus of elasticity (Figs. 23 and 24) [27]. The color scale in SWE is usually between 0 and 180 kPa [28], and while the softest tissues are coded

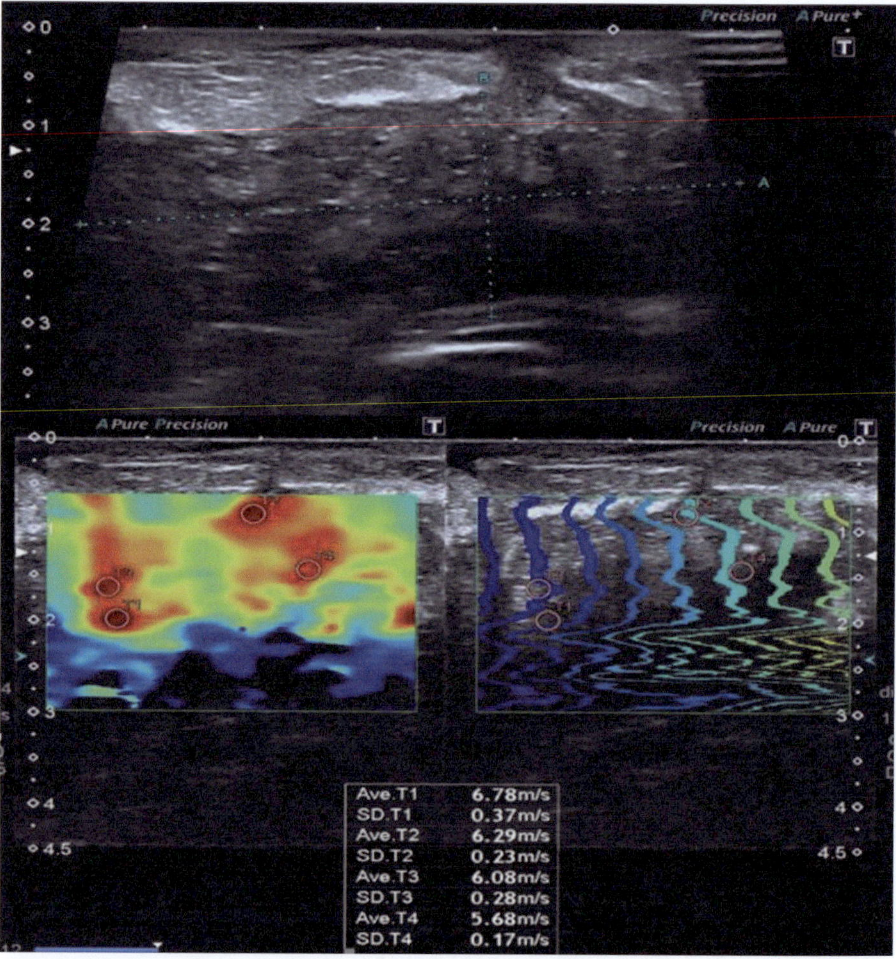

Fig. 23 A 35-year-old woman with IGM. In the grayscale examination, a large heterogeneous hypoechoic lesion in an orientation parallel to the skin is observed. In the SWE examination, the m/s measurements (6.78–5.68 m/s) are observed in the areas coded in red

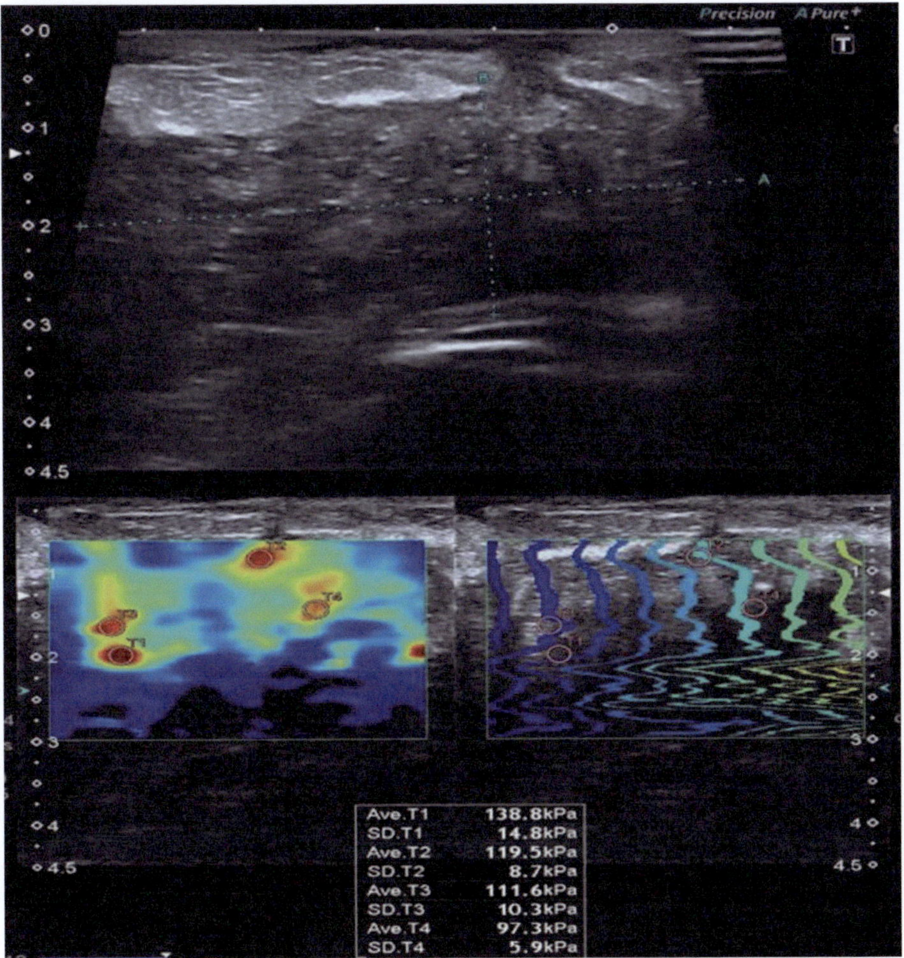

Fig. 24 A 35-year-old woman with IGM. In the grayscale examination, a large heterogeneous hypoechoic lesion in an orientation parallel to the skin is observed. In the SWE examination, the kPa measurements (138–97 kPa) are observed in the areas coded in red

in blue, the hardest tissues are coded in red. The strain values of simple cysts, adipose tissue, and dense breast tissue are 0 kPa, between 5 and 10 kPa, and 45 kPa, respectively, and the strain values of benign lesions are below 80 kPa (Fig. 25) [29]. On the other hand, benign lesions such as IGM usually tend to be harder than the normal breast tissue but softer than the malignant lesions.

A recent study has revealed that the cutoff SWV value was defined to be 4.1 m/s, where the sensitivity, specificity, positive predictive value, negative predictive value, and accuracy for diagnosing malignancies were 97.5%, 93%, 92.6%, 97.6%, and 95.2%, respectively [30]. The findings in the study by Makal and Güvenç [30] demonstrated that unnecessary biopsies could be prevented using this procedure. Even

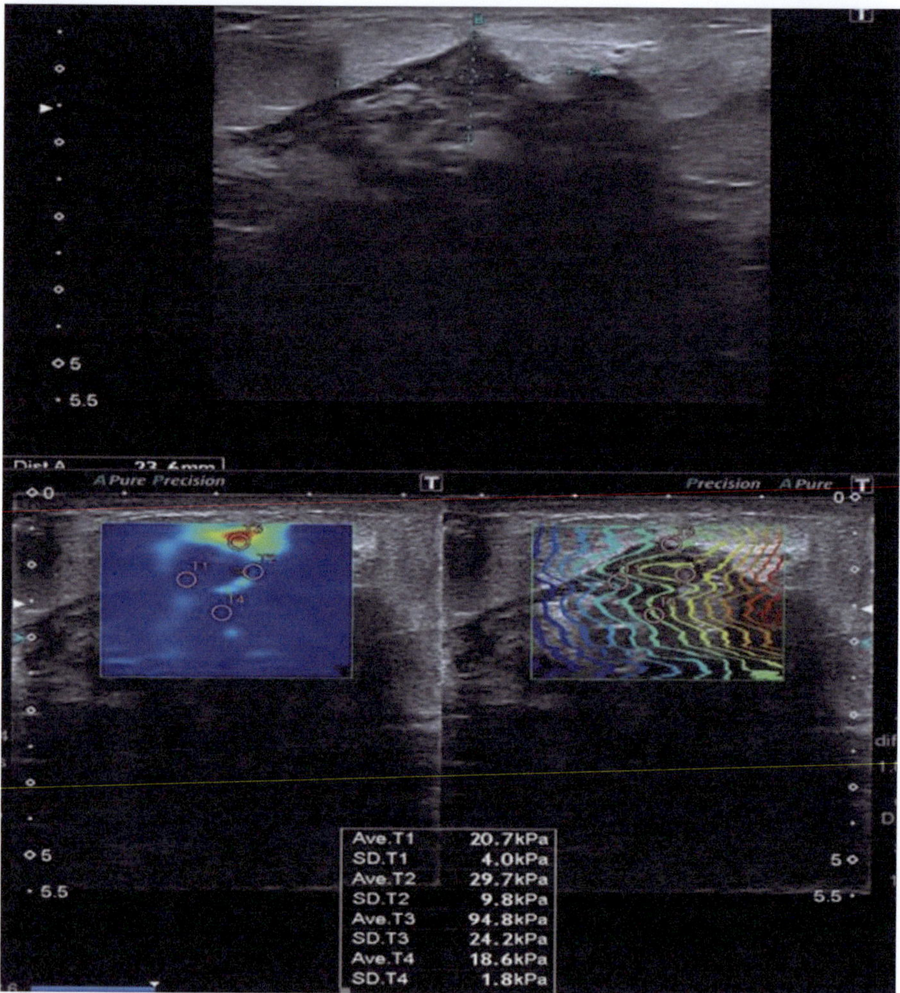

Fig. 25 A 28-year-old woman with IGM. In the grayscale examination, a hypoechoic mass with irregular contours is observed. In the SWE examination, the measurements are observed in the area coded in red (94 kPa) and in the areas coded in blue (18,20, 29 kPa)

though the BI-RADS score was found to be higher, the SWV and SWE scores were detected to be lower in those with IGM. Both BI-RADS and SWE scores were determined to be significantly higher in those with breast cancers. It is a fact that stiff lesions appear larger on elastography than those on the conventional US owing to the desmoplastic reaction around the lesion. However, no association was detected between the SWV values and the size of the lesions [30].

In several studies, it is stated that lesions evaluated as the BI-RADS 4A category will be downgraded to BI-RADS 3, and the BI-RADS 3 lesions can be upgraded to the BI-RADS 4 category according to the reassessments using US elastography [18,

30–34]. Evaluations with BI-RADS 4 category are likely to cover numerous malignancies ranging from 2% to 95%. Most of the recommended biopsies are related to the BI-RADS 4 category; therefore, studies should primarily aim at BI-RADS 4 lesions to determine breast cancers at an early stage. In conventional US, low PPVs are more related to BI-RADS 4 lesions, and so they lead to an increased number of unnecessary biopsies. In the study carried out by Memis et al. [2], when SWV values were added, and the cutoff was set as 4.08 m/s, the sensitivity, specificity, and accuracy of BI-RADS 4 lesions were 87.2%, 86.7%, and 87% in the diagnosis of malignancies, respectively [10]. In conclusion, SWE is a method with higher sensitivity and specificity in differentiating IGM and breast cancers with lower SWV and SWE scores [30].

When compared with benign inflammatory lymph nodes, metastatic axillary lymph nodes are more vascular and harder. Choi et al. [35] investigated axillary lymph nodes and reported that when the B-mode US and elastography were combined in practice, the best diagnostic performance was achieved with a sensitivity rate of 87%.

3   Interventional Procedures

Percutaneous needle biopsies are now the standard approach as an alternative to open surgical biopsy in the pathological diagnosis of suspicious lesions detected through breast imaging methods.

US, mammography, or MRI can be utilized to guide interventional procedures in the breast. The guiding method should be chosen depending on the accessibility and visibility of the lesion, the effectiveness of the technique, easiness in positioning the patient, and the practitioner's experience. The method by which the best image of the lesion is obtained should be preferred. The stereotactic method is so effective in the identification of the lesions observed in mammography, especially in sampling microcalcifications. The stereotactic method can be conducted in the units having a prone table or where mammography is added to the method in the settings. US guidance provides an advantage for detecting the lesions due to features such as easy approach, absence of ionizing radiation, real-time imaging, and its fast and easy practicability. Suspicious axillary lymph nodes are also likely to be sampled easily under US guidance. US-guided fine-needle aspiration (FNAB) and core-needle biopsies, whether used to aspirate fluid collections or not, are widespread modalities utilized in diagnosing IGM. Even though FNAB may be beneficial initially in distinguishing between inflammatory, benign breast conditions, and malignancies, the definitive diagnosis should histopathologically be confirmed by using a core-needle, vacuum-assisted, or surgical biopsy. In a study by Kok and Telisinghe [36], 23 patients with IGM initially underwent FNAB and their diagnosis was confirmed using core-needle and/or surgical biopsy. FNAB was reported to be useful in the diagnosis in only four of 24 IGM lesions. The use of a large needle gauge biopsy provides a more accurate result. By using long-throw (2-cm) 14G caliber needles in the core-needle biopsy, the most sufficient specimen can be obtained with a fully automatic biopsy gun. However, in vacuum biopsy, 8–11G caliber needles are used, and since the amount of specimen obtained in a vacuum biopsy is greater, the cases are less likely to be underdiagnosed. In microcalcification and structural distortion, vacuum biopsy also provides higher sensitivity and specificity compared with core biopsy. Even so, a core biopsy using a 14G caliber needle is sufficient for other types of lesions.

Because of significant scratching, absence of breast symmetry, deformities in breasts, and the possibility of unhealed ulcers or sinus tract formations, diagnostic excisional biopsies are unwanted in IGM lesions. Sampling procedure from the thick walls of the necrotic lesions or abscesses and specimens of inflamed areas including vascular signals may yield adequate pathological results [12, 13].

4   Breast Magnetic Resonance Imaging

MRI is a highly specific and sensitive modality for detecting lesions in inflammatory pathologies of the breast and evaluating the extent of such pathologies [4]. Although the asymmetrical density is observed on mammography, the lesion may not be detected on sonography in some cases. In addition to the dense character of the breast parenchyma especially in young patients, MRI has an advantage of detecting lesions that cannot be monitored by US or mammography due to the edema in the surrounding tissues [4].

Idiopathic granulomatous mastitis is a frequent challenge among premenopausal women exhibiting the signs of mastitis and masses. Thus, IGM should be initially evaluated on US, apart from mammography and MRI. The therapeutic approach recommended is rapidly administered antibiotic therapy and monitoring of patient on admission. The monitoring process and response to the treatment should be followed up via US. MRI can also be used for the follow-up in aggressive, diffuse, and irresponsive diseases. MRI may be beneficial in the assessment of possible residual disease after treatment or in monitoring patients receiving conservative treatment. BI-RADS is a risk assessment and quality assurance tool providing an effective standardization in reporting routine breast US and mammography and is also so useful in guiding MRI examinations. When a mass lesion or contrast enhancement is not present, the finding is categorized as smooth margins, non-enhancing internal septations, and a persistent type of enhancement is categorized as the BI-RADS 2 category (benign). Focal masses with a round, oval, or macrolobular shape, smooth margins and a persistent or plateau time course, and asymmetric, non-mass enhancements of focal or regional distribution are categorized as BI-RADS 3 (probably benign). However, the lesions with suspicious morphology (for masses with an irregular shape, irregular or spiculated margins, and heterogeneous or rim enhancement and for non-mass lesions with especially clumped and dendritic-type enhancement at ductal and segmental distribution) or rapid washout time course are categorized as BI-RADS 4 (suspicious findings), while those with suspicious morphology, more than 90% wash-in rate, and plateau or rapid washout time course are categorized as BI-RADS 5 (probably malignant) [37].

It has been reported that MRI is required for the optimal BI-RADS classification of the lesions and the exclusion of malignancy in a large series. In a study, the diagnosis through BI-RADS 3 category was obtained significantly higher with MRI examination (82.75%), compared with other conventional methods (55.17%) [4].

Although IGM is a disease displaying mostly a unilateral distribution, MRI is known as a particularly significant imaging modality in revealing the extent of the lesion and the contralateral breast involvement. In a previous study, the prevalence rates of peripheral, subareolar, and diffuse IGM lesions have been reported as 50%, 25%, and 25%, respectively [38, 39].

Although MRI findings vary depending on the severity of inflammation in IGM, the most common finding is the increase in focal or diffuse asymmetric signals without displaying a mass effect (Fig. 26). Single or multiple, split or combined peripheral ring-enhancing abscesses of different sizes are among the frequently encountered MRI findings (Fig. 27) [4]. In advanced cases, large fluid collections with or without skin openings can be observed in the abnormally enhanced parenchyma (Fig. 28). Thickening of the breast skin and nipple retraction are also among the first remarkable findings of IGM which have been noticed on MRI, compared with other investigation methods (Fig. 29). MRI changes consistent with necrosis or abscesses, fistula tracts, dilated ductal structures with enhanced walls, and lymphadenopathy are among other findings observed on MRI (Fig. 30). Various tiny lesions displaying confluent or well-defined borders, T2 hyperintensity, and rim enhancement on MRI have been considered to represent micro-abscesses (Fig. 31) [5]. IGM is generally observed as segmental/regional non-mass enhancement areas and peripherally contrasted mass lesions during the contrast-enhanced examination (Figs. 32 and 33). The affected parenchymal area and adjacent surrounding tissues show more contrast enhancement than normal tissues, independently of the dynamic contrast enhancement (Figs. 30, 32, and 33) [40].

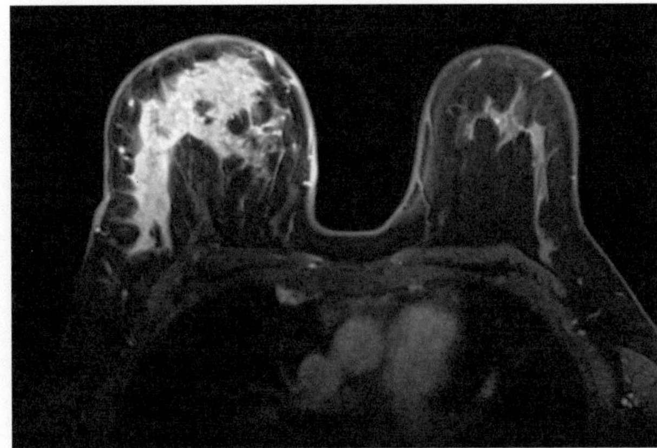

Fig. 26 A 36-year-old woman with IGM. Asymmetric regional enhancement in the outer quadrant of the right breast on the transverse contrast-enhanced fat saturation (fat-sat) T1-weighted image

Fig. 27 A 30-year-old woman with IGM. In the right breast in the outer quadrant and retroareolar region, multiple abscesses with peripheral enhancement and asymmetric regional enhancement on the transverse contrast-enhanced fat-sat T1-weighted image

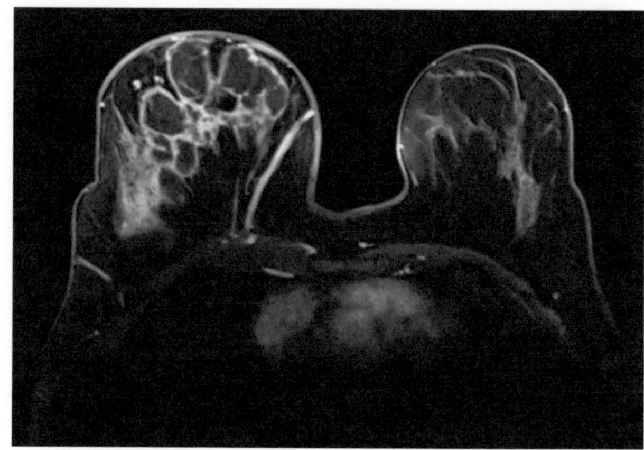

Fig. 28 A 31-year-old woman with IGM. Diffuse edema in the outer quadrant of the right breast, thickening of the periareolar skin, and hyperintense abscess in the retroareolar region on the transverse fat-sat T2-weighted image

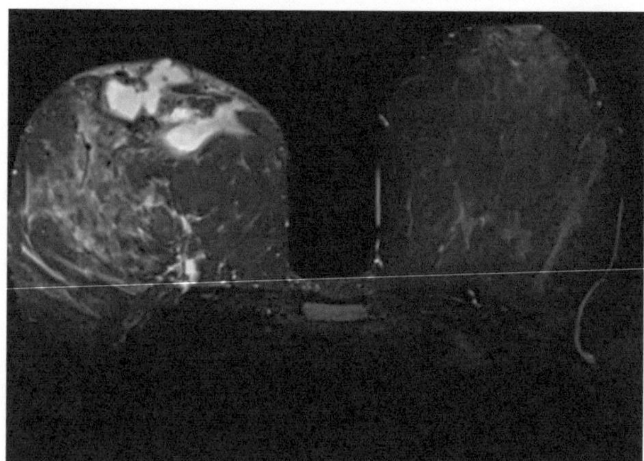

Fig. 29 A 30-year-old woman with IGM. Thickening of the skin in the inner quadrant of the right breast, nipple retraction, and retroareolar enhancement are seen on the transverse contrast-enhanced fat-sat T1-weighted image

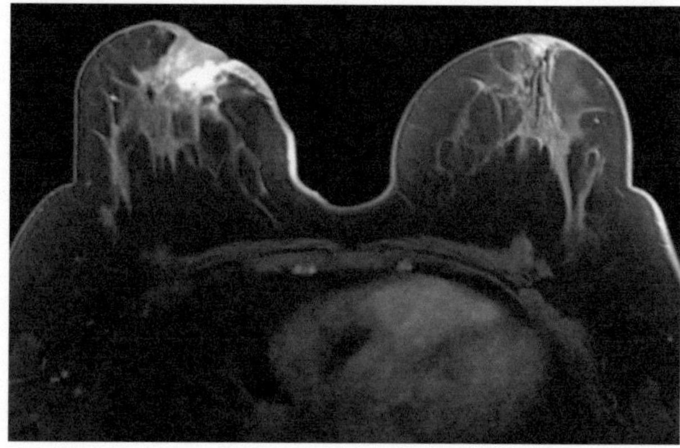

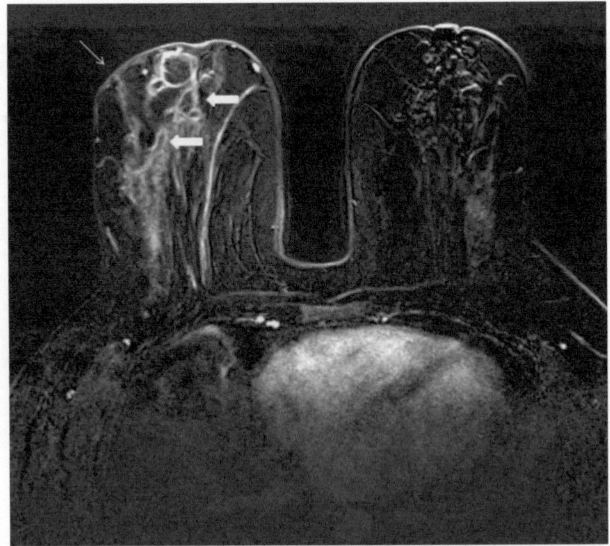

Fig. 30 A 38-year-old woman with IGM. Transverse subtraction T1 image shows asymmetric regional enhancement in the outer quadrant of the right breast, skin fistulization in the outer quadrant (thin arrow), and enhanced tubular connections (thick arrows)

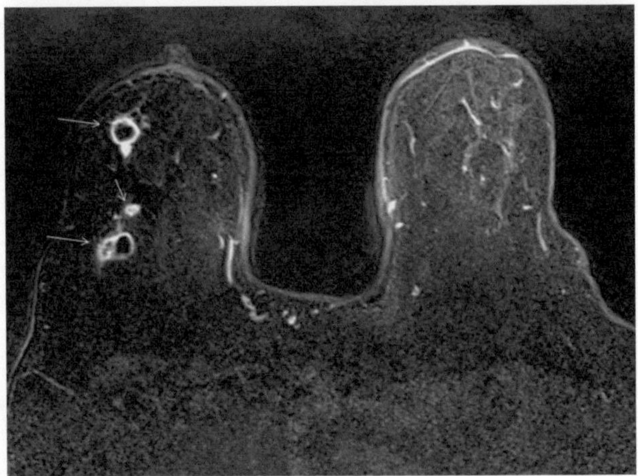

Fig. 31 A 35-year-old woman with IGM. Transverse subtraction T1 image shows micro-abscesses with peripheral enhancement (arrows)

Dynamic MRI investigations are beneficial in the differentiation of malignant and benign lesions by determining the kinetic properties of the lesion as a contribution to the morphological characteristics through series obtained after the injection of the contrast agent.

The dynamic data are correlated with alterations in the vascularization and pathophysiological structure of the tissue and based on the principle that those alterations are different between malignant and benign lesions. While malignant lesions are expected to have faster and more pronounced enhancement and washing, the contrast enhancement of benign lesions is expected to be slow and to continue persistently. However, the early contrast enhancement can vary in both malignant and

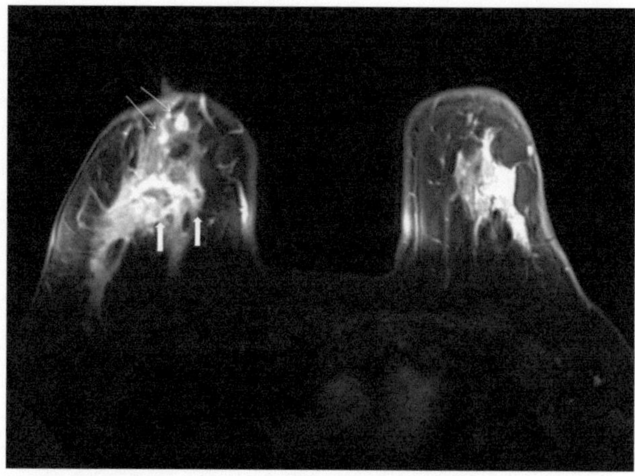

Fig. 32 A 29-year-old woman with IGM. Axial T1-weighted, fat-sat, contrast-enhanced MR images show asymmetric regional enhancement in the outer quadrant, nodular enhancements in the retroareolar region (thin arrows), and micro-abscesses with peripheral enhancement (thick arrows) in the right breast

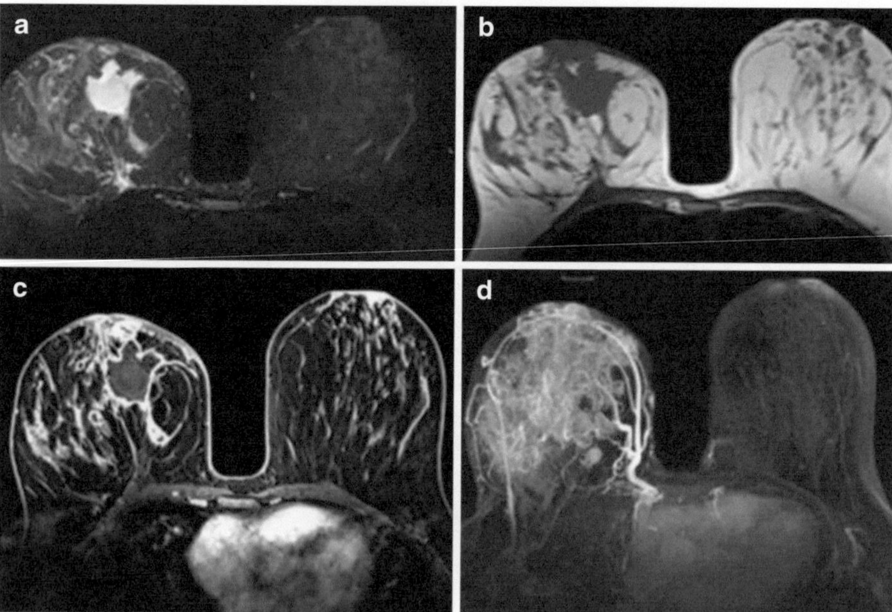

Fig. 33 A 31-year-old woman with IGM. Breast abscess on transverse images. T2 fat-sat image (**a**) shows regional edema in the outer quadrant of the right breast and a hyperintense lesion with lobulated contours. The abscess is seen hypointense on T1 image (**b**) and peripheral enhancement on contrast-enhanced T1 image (**c**). Significant diffuse enhancement in the right breast is observed on maximal intensity projection (MIP) image (**d**)

benign lesions [41, 42]. Following the administration of contrast agent, three possible enhancement curves related to time intensity are observed for a breast lesion on MRI; in the course of the curve within the mid-to-late period, while a type 1 curve pattern is mostly seen in benign lesions (Fig. 34), type 2–3 curve patterns are present in malignant lesions (Figs. 35 and 36) [41]. A recent study in IGM patients has also revealed that as a result of kinetic analyses of non-mass-like contrast-enhanced areas, lesions, and lesion walls, type 1 kinetic curves were seen in 24 (82.7%) patients at all levels, type 2 kinetic curves in the lesion walls in four (13.8%) patients, and type 3 kinetic curves in the lesion walls and non-mass-like contrast-enhanced areas in one patient (3.4%) [4]. The kinetic analysis may have additional contributions to differentiating benign lesions from malignancy in IGM patients where the mass-like lesion without prominent inflammatory findings is seen in the foreground.

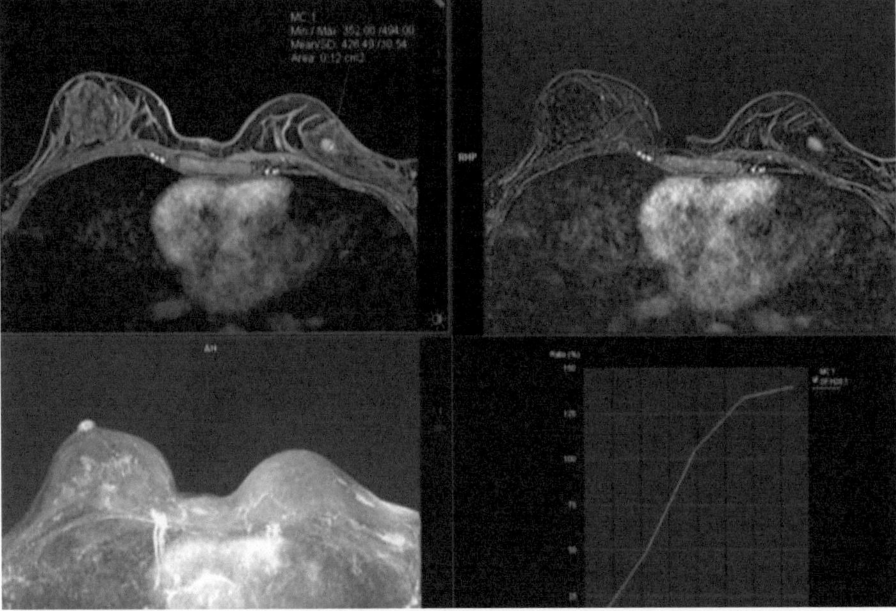

Fig. 34 A 24-year-old woman with fibroadenoma. The round mass in the upper outer quadrant of the left breast has a type 1 curve pattern on dynamic review

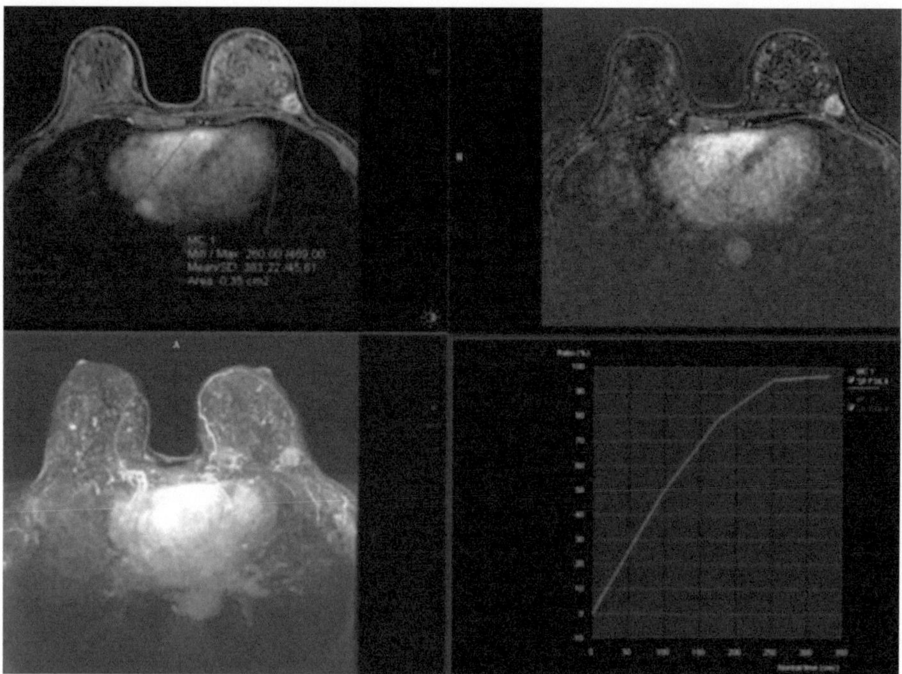

Fig. 35 A 29-year-old woman. The round mass in the outer quadrant of the left breast has a type 2 curve pattern on dynamic review

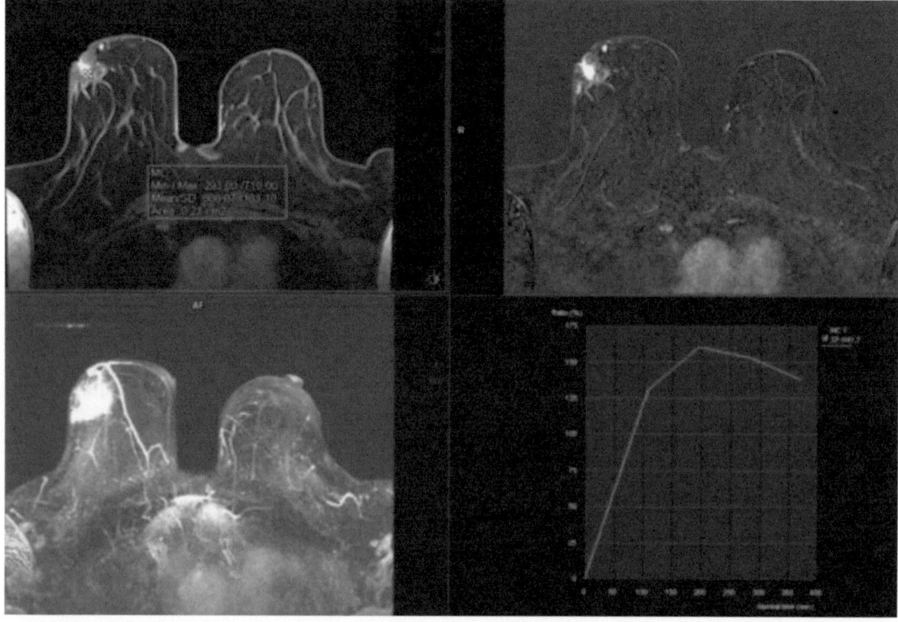

Fig. 36 Breast carcinoma. Axial images show enhanced mass with irregular borders. The mass has a type 3 curve pattern on dynamic review

4.1 Diffusion Breast Magnetic Resonance Imaging

Breast MRI has gained considerable clinical importance in recent years. The sensitivity of breast MRI examination, especially in the detection of cancer, ranges between 94% and 100% [43, 44]. However, the specificity of breast MRI is below these values in distinguishing the characteristic features of benign and malignant lesions [45, 46]. Due to the contributions to the differential diagnosis of the lesion along with the morphological and kinetic features in breast MRI, many researchers also emphasize the importance of the features of diffusion-weighted imaging (DWI) [12, 13, 45, 47]. Diffusion-weighted MRI (DW-MRI) is a non-contrast modality used to measure the motion of water particles in vivo and to analyze the microscopic nature of tissues, such as cellularity, membrane integrity, viscosity, fibers, tubules, organelles, and macromolecules. Diffusion developing in individual voxels is calculated using different DWI images, resulting in a quantitative apparent diffusion coefficient (ADC) map. DWI with quantitative ADC values have been stated to be a reliable tool in differentiating between malignant and benign breast lesions [48].

Lower ADCs are present in malignant lesions due to high cellular proliferation and the limited size of the extracellular matrix. In DWI, IGM-like inflammatory processes can reveal diffusion changes developing due to edema, inflammatory cell migration, and cellular debris. Since the necrosis of the abscess has cellular debris and high viscosity, diffusion restriction is seen at the center of the abscess (Figs. 37 and 38). In the involved parenchyma of those with IGM, restricted diffusion is seen in the majority of cases having consistently lower mean ADCs

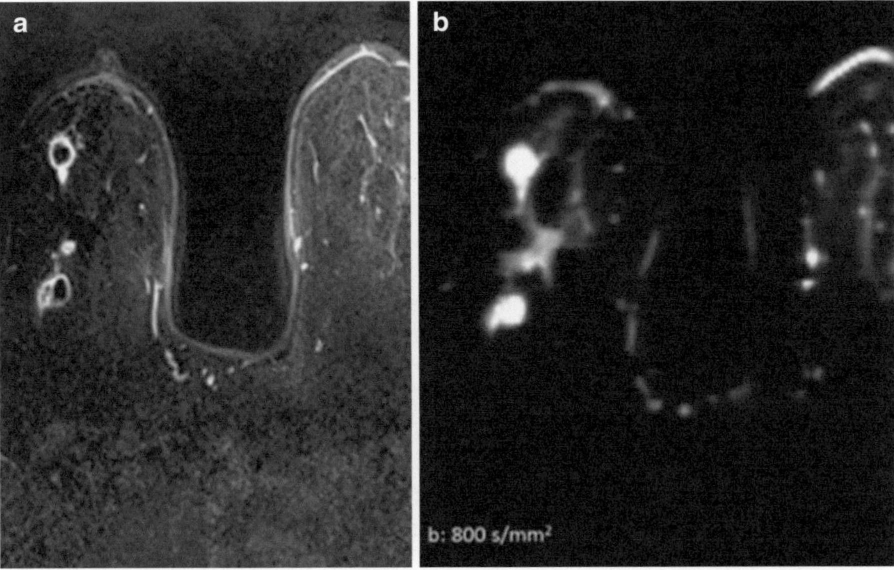

Fig. 37 Breast abscess in a patient with IGM. Subtraction axial image (**a**) shows the peripherally enhanced lesions in the right breast. Diffusion-weighted image (**b**) demonstrates diffusion restriction

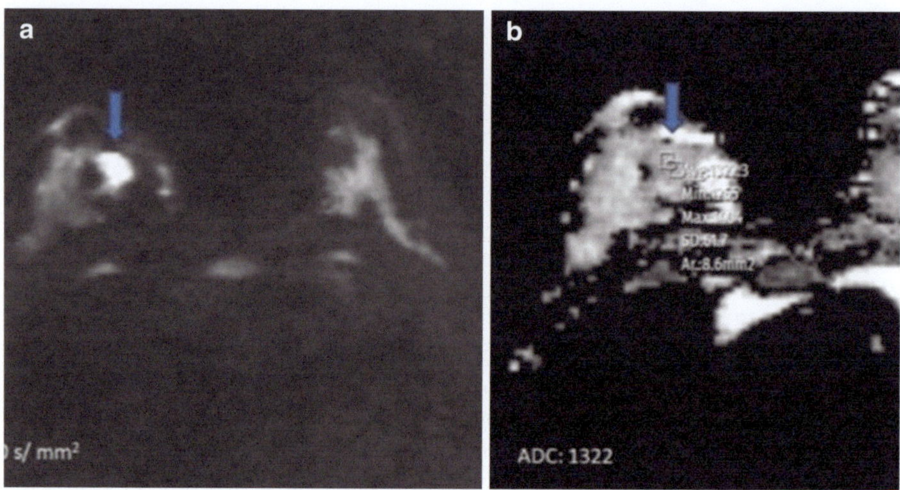

Fig. 38 Breast abscess in a patient with IGM (arrow). Diffusion-weighted image (**b**: 800 s/mm²) (**a**) demonstrates diffusion restriction. The ADC value (**b**) obtained from the center of necrosis

(1.0 × 10–3 mm²/s) than that observed for normal breast parenchyma (2.3 × 10–3 mm²/s) [40].

Baltzer et al. [49] stated that a combination of DWI and T2-weighted turbo spin echo (TSE) is capable of accurately differentiating benign mass lesions from malignancy in the breast, presenting with equal sensitivity and specificity levels without the requirement for injecting contrast material [49].

5 Positron Emission Tomography and Computed Tomography Scans (PET/CT)

To diagnose the primary breast lesions, the imaging is primarily performed by mammography, US, and MRI. In those having any known breast carcinoma, fluoro-deoxyglucose (FDG)-PET/CT is carried out to detect the unsuspected extra-axillary lymph nodes, distant metastases, and responses to the treatment. In addition, FDG-PET/CT may also provide an additional contribution to the exclusion of malignancy in suspected IGM cases, such as inflammatory breast cancer. Based on the principle of measuring the increase of glucose metabolism in malignant tumors, PET is frequently used to evaluate breast cancers. PET can be used alone or in combination with CT and/or FDG.

Hypermetabolic incidental breast lesions on FDG PET/CT are manifested in 0.36–1.12% of female patients and the prevalence of malignancies is nearly 27% to 38% [50, 51]. Further research covering a wide range of hypermetabolic breast lesions on FDG-PET/CT is required for clinicians to report FDG-PET/CT findings accurately. Considering the importance of FDG-PET imaging in detecting malignant tumors, the increased metabolic activity in oncological cells always plays a key role.

Activated inflammatory cells, including neutrophils and macrophages, increase the expression of glucose transporters as led by malignant cells, and such an increase results in trapping of the intravenous administration of FDG [52].

Increased FDG uptake in acute and chronic mastitis led by bacteria, viruses, parasites, tuberculosis, siliconoma, and surgical interventions are stated in the literature [53–55] . In patients with acute mastitis, diffuse FDG uptake can be possibly detected. As well as focal FDG uptake generally being revealed by chronic lesions, inflammatory breast carcinomas also show diffuse or focal FDG uptake in the large breasts with increased skin FDG uptake [32]. Differential diagnosis of patients with hypermetabolic breast lesions on FDG PET/CT should be investigated with other imaging studies and histopathological examination.

Acknowledgments We would like to thank Dr. E. Uysal for her support in images.

References

1. Engin G, Acunaş G, Acunaş B. Granulomatous mastitis: gray-scale and color Doppler sonographic findings. J Clin Ultrasound. 1999;27:101–6. https://doi.org/10.1002/(sici)1097-0096 (199903/04)27:3<101::aid-jcu1>3.0.co;2-i.
2. Memis A, Bilgen I, Ustun EE, Ozdemir N, Erhan Y, Kapkac M. Granulomatous mastitis: imaging findings with histopathologic correlation. Clin Radiol. 2002;57:1001–6. https://doi.org/10.1053/crad.2002.1056.
3. Yildiz S, Aralasmak A, Kadioglu H, Toprak H, Yetis H, Gucin Z, et al. Radiologic findings of idiopathic granulomatous mastitis. Med Ultrason. 2015;17:39–44. https://doi.org/10.11152/mu.2013.2066.171.rfm.
4. Oztekin PS, Durhan G, Nercis Kosar P, Erel S, Hucumenoglu S. Imaging findings in patients with granulomatous mastitis. Iran J Radiol. 2016;13:e33900. https://doi.org/10.5812/iranjradiol.33900.
5. Fazzio RT, Shah SS, Sandhu NP, Glazebrook KN. Idiopathic granulomatous mastitis: imaging update and review. Insights Imaging. 2016;7:531–9. https://doi.org/10.1007/s13244-016-0499-0.
6. Pluguez-Turull CW, Nanyes JE, Quintero CJ, Alizai H, Mais DD, Kist KA, et al. Idiopathic granulomatous mastitis: manifestations at multimodality imaging and pitfalls. Radiographics. 2018;38:330–56. https://doi.org/10.1148/rg.2018170095.
7. Sabaté JM, Clotet M, Gómez A, De Las HP, Torrubia S, Salinas T. Radiologic evaluation of uncommon inflammatory and reactive breast disorders. Radiographics. 2005;25:411–24. https://doi.org/10.1148/rg.252045077.
8. D'Orsi CJ, Sickles EA, Mendelson EB, et al. ACR BI-RADS® atlas, breast imaging reporting and data system. Reston, VA: American College of Radiology; 2013.
9. Cho SH, Park SH. Mimickers of breast malignancy on breast sonography. J Ultrasound Med. 2013;32:2029–36. https://doi.org/10.7863/ultra.32.11.2029.
10. Teke M, Teke F, Alan B, Türkoğlu A, Hamidi C, Göya C, et al. Differential diagnosis of idiopathic granulomatous mastitis and breast cancer using acoustic radiation force impulse imaging. J Med Ultrason (2001). 2017;44:109–15. https://doi.org/10.1007/s10396-016-0749-2.
11. Toprak N, Gunduz AM. Idiopathic granulomatous mastitis and other types of mastitis; comparison of ultrasound findings. East J Med. 2021;26:339–43. https://doi.org/10.5505/ejm.2021.81598.
12. Durur-Subasi I. Diagnostic and interventional radiology in idiopathic granulomatous mastitis. Eurasian J Med. 2019a;51:293–7. https://doi.org/10.5152/eurasianjmed.2019.19211.

13. Durur-Subasi I. DW-MRI of the breast: a pictorial review. Insights Imaging. 2019b;10:61. https://doi.org/10.1186/s13244-019-0745-3.
14. Barr RG, Destounis S, Lackey LB 2nd, Svensson WE, Balleyguier C, Smith C. Evaluation of breast lesions using sonographic elasticity imaging: a multicenter trial. J Ultrasound Med. 2012;31:281–7. https://doi.org/10.7863/jum.2012.31.2.281.
15. Krouskop TA, Wheeler TM, Kallel F, Garra BS, Hall T. Elastic moduli of breast and prostate tissues under compression. Ultrason Imaging. 1998;20:260–74. https://doi.org/10.1177/016173469802000403.
16. Ueno E, Umemoto T, Bando H, Tohno E, Waki K, Matsumura T. New quantitative method in breast elastography: fat lesion ratio (FLR). Radiological Society of North America 2007 Scientific Assembly and Annual Meeting, November 25–November 30, Chicago IL. 2007. http://archive.rsna.org/2007/5015476.html.
17. Itoh A, Ueno E, Tohno E, Kamma H, Takahashi H, Shiina T, et al. Breast disease: clinical application of US elastography for diagnosis. Radiology. 2006;239:341–50. https://doi.org/10.1148/radiol.2391041676.
18. Barr RG, Nakashima K, Amy D, Cosgrove D, Farrokh A, Schafer F, et al. WFUMB guidelines and recommendations for clinical use of ultrasound elastography: part 2: breast. Ultrasound Med Biol. 2015;41:1148–60. https://doi.org/10.1016/j.ultrasmedbio.2015.03.008.
19. Gong X, Xu Q, Xu Z, Xiong P, Yan W, Chen Y. Real-time elastography for the differentiation of benign and malignant breast lesions: a meta-analysis. Breast Cancer Res Treat. 2011;130:11–8. https://doi.org/10.1007/s10549-011-1745-2.
20. Ginat DT, Destounis SV, Barr RG, Castaneda B, Strang JG, Rubens DJ. US elastography of breast and prostate lesions. Radiographics. 2009;29:2007–16. https://doi.org/10.1148/rg.297095058.
21. Barr RG. Real-time ultrasound elasticity of the breast: initial clinical results. Ultrasound Q. 2010;26:61–6. https://doi.org/10.1097/RUQ.0b013e3181dc7ce4.
22. Ricci P, Maggini E, Mancuso E, Lodise P, Cantisani V, Catalano C. Clinical application of breast elastography: state of the art. Eur J Radiol. 2014;83:429–37. https://doi.org/10.1016/j.ejrad.2013.05.007.
23. Alhabshi SM, Rahmat K, Abdul Halim N, Aziz S, Radhika S, Gan GC, et al. Semi-quantitative and qualitative assessment of breast ultrasound elastography in differentiating between malignant and benign lesions. Ultrasound Med Biol. 2013;39:568–78. https://doi.org/10.1016/j.ultrasmedbio.2012.10.016.
24. Cho N, Moon WK, Kim HY, Chang JM, Park SH, Lyou CY. Sonoelastographic strain index for differentiation of benign and malignant nonpalpable breast masses. J Ultrasound Med. 2010;29:1–7. https://doi.org/10.7863/jum.2010.29.1.1.
25. Thomas A, Degenhardt F, Farrokh A, Wojcinski S, Slowinski T, Fischer T. Significant differentiation of focal breast lesions: calculation of strain ratio in breast sonoelastography. Acad Radiol. 2010;17:558–63. https://doi.org/10.1016/j.acra.2009.12.006.
26. Cindil E, Gultekin S. Meme elastografisi. Türk Radyoloji Seminerleri Trd Sem. 2019;7:50–62. https://doi.org/10.5152/trs.2019.712.
27. Cosgrove DO, Berg WA, Doré CJ, Skyba DM, Henry JP, Gay J, et al. Shear wave elastography for breast masses is highly reproducible. Eur Radiol. 2012;22:1023–32. https://doi.org/10.1007/s00330-011-2340-y.
28. Chen L, He J, Liu G, Shao K, Zhou M, Li B, Chen X. Diagnostic performances of shear-wave elastography for identification of malignant breast lesions: a meta-analysis. Jpn J Radiol. 2014;32(10):592–9. https://doi.org/10.1007/s11604-014-0349-2. Epub 2014 Sep 7. PMID: 25195123.
29. Barr RG. Shear wave imaging of the breast: still on the learning curve. J Ultrasound Med. 2012;31:347–50. https://doi.org/10.7863/jum.2012.31.3.347.
30. Makal GB, Güvenç İ. The role of shear wave elastography in differentiating idiopathic granulomatous mastitis from breast cancer. Acad Radiol. 2021;28:339–44. https://doi.org/10.1016/j.acra.2020.02.008.

31. Feldmann A, Langlois C, Dewailly M, Martinez EF, Boulanger L, Kerdraon O, et al. Shear wave elastography (SWE): an analysis of breast lesion characterization in 83 breast lesions. Ultrasound Med Biol. 2015;41:2594–604. https://doi.org/10.1016/j.ultrasmedbio.2015.05.019.

32. Yang WT, Le-Petross HT, Macapinlac H, Carkaci S, Gonzalez-Angulo AM, Dawood S, et al. Inflammatory breast cancer: PET/CT, MRI, mammography, and sonography findings. Breast Cancer Res Treat. 2008;109:417–26. https://doi.org/10.1007/s10549-007-9671-z.

33. Yi A, Cho N, Chang JM, Koo HR, La Yun B, Moon WK. Sonoelastography for 1,786 non-palpable breast masses: diagnostic value in the decision to biopsy. Eur Radiol. 2012;22:1033–40. https://doi.org/10.1007/s00330-011-2341-x.

34. Youk JH, Gweon HM, Son EJ, Han KH, Kim JA. Diagnostic value of commercially available shear-wave elastography for breast cancers: integration into BI-RADS classification with subcategories of category 4. Eur Radiol. 2013;23:2695–704. https://doi.org/10.1007/s00330-013-2873-3.

35. Choi JJ, Kang BJ, Kim SH, Lee JH, Jeong SH, Yim HW, et al. Role of sonographic elastography in the differential diagnosis of axillary lymph nodes in breast cancer. J Ultrasound Med. 2011;30:429–36. https://doi.org/10.7863/jum.2011.30.4.429.

36. Kok KY, Telisinghe PU. Granulomatous mastitis: presentation, treatment and outcome in 43 patients. Surgeon. 2010;8:197–201. https://doi.org/10.1016/j.surge.2010.02.002.

37. Kul S, Cansu A, Alhan E, Dinc H, Gunes G, Reis A. Contribution of diffusion-weighted imaging to dynamic contrast-enhanced MRI in the characterization of breast tumors. AJR Am J Roentgenol. 2011;196:210–7. https://doi.org/10.2214/AJR.10.4258.

38. Hovanessian Larsen LJ, Peyvandi B, Klipfel N, Grant E, Iyengar G. Granulomatous lobular mastitis: imaging, diagnosis, and treatment. AJR Am J Roentgenol. 2009;193:574–81. https://doi.org/10.2214/AJR.08.1528.

39. Lee JH, Oh KK, Kim EK, Kwack KS, Jung WH, Lee HK. Radiologic and clinical features of idiopathic granulomatous lobular mastitis mimicking advanced breast cancer. Yonsei Med J. 2006;47:78–84. https://doi.org/10.3349/ymj.2006.47.1.78.

40. Manogna P, Bhawna Dev B, Joseph LD, Ramakrishnan R. Idiopathic granulomatous mastitis—our experience. Egypt J Radiol Nucl Med. 2020;51:15. https://doi.org/10.1186/s43055-019-0126-4.

41. Aksoy DO, Kilicoglu ZG, Yilmaz G, Kadioglu E, Telli S, Simşek MM. Comparison of morphological and kinetic parameters in distinction of benign and malignant breast lesions in dynamic contrast enhanced magnetic resonance imaging. Dicle Med J. 2013;40:562–9. https://doi.org/10.5798/diclemedj.0921.2013.04.0333.

42. Schnall MD, Blume J, Bluemke DA, DeAngelis GA, DeBruhl N, Harms S, et al. Diagnostic architectural and dynamic features at breast MR imaging: multicenter study. Radiology. 2006;238:42–53. https://doi.org/10.1148/radiol.2381042117.

43. Mahoney MC, Gatsonis C, Hanna L, DeMartini WB, Lehman C. Positive predictive value of BI-RADS MR imaging. Radiology. 2012;264:51–8. https://doi.org/10.1148/radiol.12110619.

44. Warren RM, Pointon L, Thompson D, Hoff R, Gilbert FJ, Padhani A, et al. Reading protocol for dynamic contrast-enhanced MR images of the breast: sensitivity and specificity analysis. Radiology. 2005;236:779–88. https://doi.org/10.1148/radiol.2363040735.

45. Bluemke DA, Gatsonis CA, Chen MH, DeAngelis GA, DeBruhl N, Harms S, et al. Magnetic resonance imaging of the breast prior to biopsy. JAMA. 2004;292:2735–42. https://doi.org/10.1001/jama.292.22.2735.

46. Wiener JI, Schilling KJ, Adami C, Obuchowski NA. Assessment of suspected breast cancer by MRI: a prospective clinical trial using a combined kinetic and morphologic analysis. AJR Am J Roentgenol. 2005;184:878–86. https://doi.org/10.2214/ajr.184.3.01840878.

47. Durur-Subasi I, Durur-Karakaya A, Karaman A, Demirci E, Alper F, Yılmazel-Ucar E, et al. Value of MRI sequences for prediction of invasive breast carcinoma size. J Med Imaging Radiat Oncol. 2014;58:565–8. https://doi.org/10.1111/1754-9485.12205.

48. Altay C, Balci P, Altay S, Karasu S, Saydam S, Canda T, Dicle O. Diffusion-weighted MR imaging: role in the differential diagnosis of breast lesions. JBR-BTR. 2014;97:211–6. https://doi.org/10.5334/jbr-btr.80.

49. Baltzer PA, Benndorf M, Dietzel M, Gajda M, Camara O, Kaiser WA. Sensitivity and specificity of unenhanced MR mammography (DWI combined with T2-weighted TSE imaging, ueMRM) for the differentiation of mass lesions. Eur Radiol. 2010;20:1101–10. https://doi.org/10.1007/s00330-009-1654-5.

50. Kang BJ, Lee JH, Yoo IR, Kim SH, Choi JJ, Jeong SH, et al. Clinical significance of incidental finding of focal activity in the breast at 18F-FDG PET/CT. AJR Am J Roentgenol. 2011;197:341–7. https://doi.org/10.2214/AJR.10.6126.

51. Lim S, Lee EH, Park JM, Chang YW, Kim HH, Jeong SH. Role of combined BI-RADS assessment using mammography and sonography for evaluation of incidental hypermetabolic lesions in the breast on 18F-FDG PET-CT. Acta Radiol. 2013;54:1117–24. https://doi.org/10.1177/0284185113492453.

52. Dong A, Wang Y, Lu J, Zuo C. Spectrum of the breast lesions with increased 18F-FDG uptake on PET/CT. Clin Nucl Med. 2016;41:543–57. https://doi.org/10.1097/RLU.0000000000001203.

53. Adejolu M, Huo L, Rohren E, Santiago L, Yang WT. False-positive lesions mimicking breast cancer on FDG PET and PET/CT. AJR Am J Roentgenol. 2012;198:W304-314. https://doi.org/10.2214/AJR.11.7130.

54. Benveniste AP, Yang W, Benveniste MF, Mawlawi OR, Marom EM. Benign breast lesions detected by positron emission tomography-computed tomography. Eur J Radiol. 2014;83:919–29. https://doi.org/10.1016/j.ejrad.2014.02.010.

55. Choi EK, Oh JK, Chung YA. Herpes zoster mimicking breast cancer with axillary lymph node metastasis on PET/CT. Clin Nucl Med. 2015;40:572–3. https://doi.org/10.1097/RLU.0000000000000804.

Imaging Appearances and Differential Diagnosis of Idiopathic Granulomatous Mastitis

Mia Morgan and William Teh

1 Introduction

Idiopathic granulomatous mastitis (IGM) is a rare, benign, inflammatory process involving chronic lobulitis of the breast parenchyma. First described by Kessler and Wolloch [1], the condition is characterized by the presence of sterile noncaseating lobulocentric granulomata in the absence of a confirmed underlying diagnosis. Despite IGM being an essentially benign entity, the disease process can follow a rather unpredictable and aggressive course with persistent or recurrent episodes necessitating surgical intervention. Radiologically, IGM can mimic many other pathologies including breast carcinoma which has, in some cases, resulted in rather radical breast surgery including mastectomy. Patients can present with suspicious clinical findings suggestive of malignancy including a palpable firm breast mass which is the most common clinical presentation of IGM [2], nipple retraction, distortion of the breast contour, and ulceration as well as sinus formation.

The location and distribution within the breast are variable with reports of involvement of the breast periphery and subareolar location as well as more diffuse involvement. The majority of cases are unilateral with bilaterality reported between 1% and 9% [2].

In this chapter we aim to provide an overview of the varied imaging appearances of IGM in the context of the broad range of differential diagnoses. We hope that this will increase awareness of this disease entity thereby reducing the risk of delayed diagnosis and inappropriate management.

M. Morgan · W. Teh (✉)
Department of Radiology, London North West University Healthcare NHS Trust, Northwick Park Hospital, London, UK

H. Koksal, N. Kadoglou (eds.), *Idiopathic Granulomatous Mastitis*,
https://doi.org/10.1007/978-3-031-30391-3_8

2 Radiological Appearances

Mammography and ultrasound (US) are the main imaging modalities in the diagnostic workup but in selected cases magnetic resonance imaging (MRI) may also add valuable information. Patients younger than 40 years of age should have ultrasound (US) scans using a high-frequency linear probe as first-line investigation with discretionary mammography if the findings are thought to be suspicious. Patients over 40 years will usually receive both mammography and US. In both age groups, mammography is only used in the absence of pregnancy or breastfeeding at the time of presentation.

Appearances can be nonspecific and there are no radiological findings that are pathognomonic of IGM. Radiological appearances are usually that of an inflammatory process with a differential diagnosis including both benign and malignant pathologies. The radiologist's role is therefore critical to the diagnostic pathway in an attempt to exclude all other pathologies before a diagnosis of IGM can be made. Given the indiscriminate radiological findings, performing an image-guided biopsy is often the cornerstone of diagnosis. Historically, a fine-needle aspirate of the affected breast parenchyma has been performed for cytology; however, this is now considered inadequate and tissue sampling with a wide-bore biopsy needle is required for histological analysis. Subsequent multidisciplinary team (MDT) discussion is paramount to ensure clinical, radiological, and pathological concordance.

Once the diagnosis of IGM has been established, imaging continues to play a vital role in the management of this disease, for determining disease extent, aiding with presurgical planning, identification of abscess formation, evaluation of treatment response, and subsequent surveillance [2].

3 Mammography

One of the most common mammographic features of IGM is that of an asymmetric density which can appear either focal or diffuse. An ill-defined mass is another frequently encountered mammographic manifestation [2] (Figs. 1a–c and 2a–d).

The breasts may be asymmetric in size with the affected side being larger, demonstrating trabecular thickening and parenchymal edema. Skin thickening, parenchymal distortion, axillary adenopathy, and nipple retraction can also be mammographic features [2, 3] (Fig. 3).

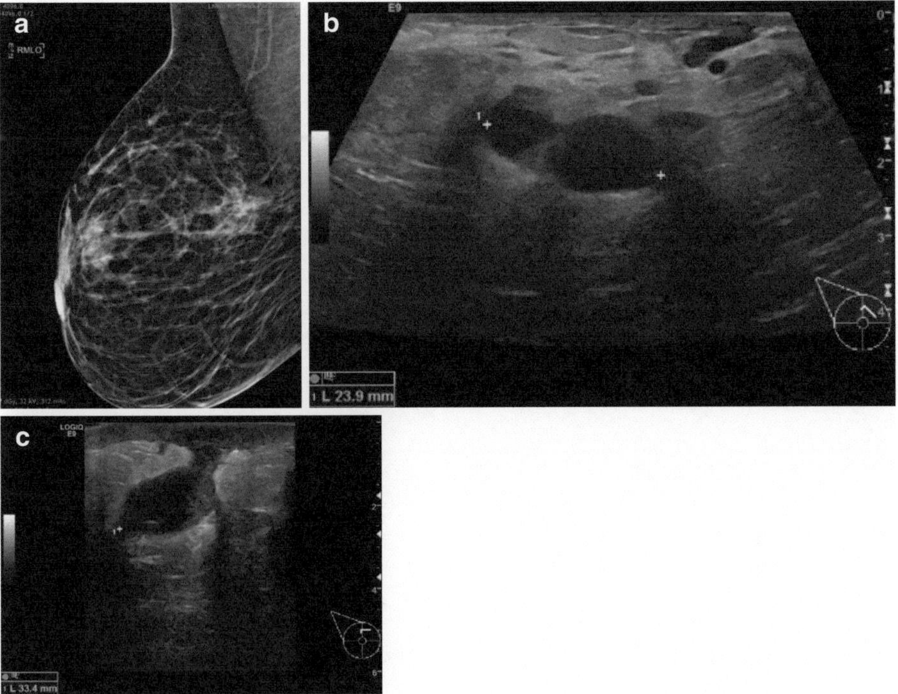

Fig. 1 (**a**) A 51-year-old woman with granulomatous mastitis. Mammograms show a right retroareolar ill-defined mass with a more posterior ill-defined asymmetry. (**b**) Ultrasound showing two focal inflammatory collections. (**c**) Retroareolar collection extending into the skin surface

Of note, inflammatory breast cancer which can present with similar clinical and imaging characteristics usually results in extensive dermal edema and inflammatory change which involves more than one-third of the breast [4]. By comparison, the dermal inflammatory change in IGM is rarely this extensive. Calcifications are an unusual radiographic feature of IGM [2]; however, segmental calcifications have occasionally been reported [5]. In some cases, mammography can appear entirely normal; however, in the case of particularly dense background glandular breast tissue or in the early stages of the disease process, a subtle mammographic abnormality can be masked.

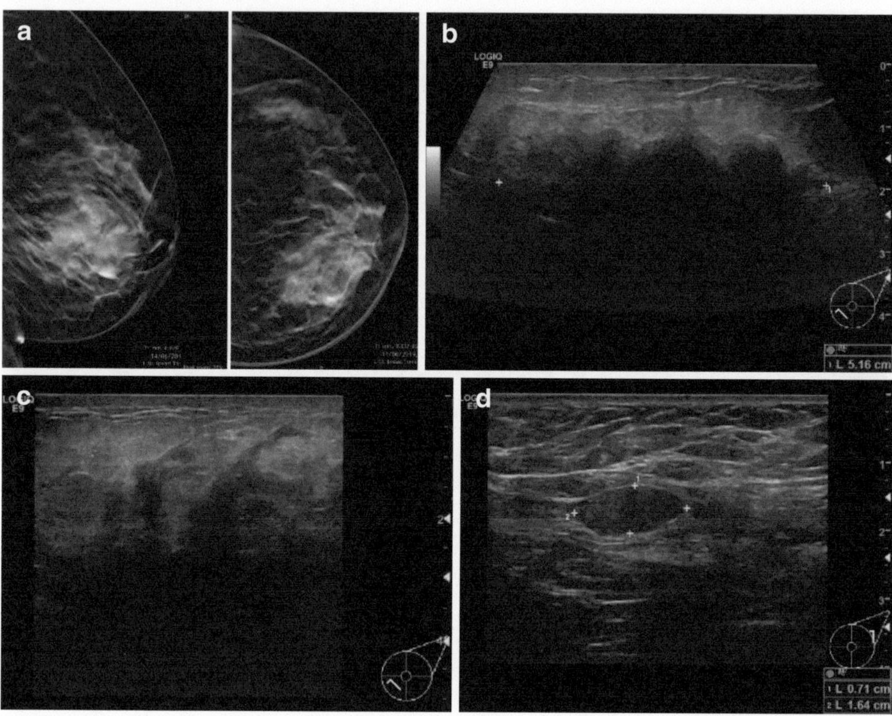

Fig. 2 (**a**) A 50-year-old woman with a firm mass in the left breast with nipple retraction suspicious for inflammatory carcinoma. Left: tomosynthesis images – there is dermal thickening and an ill-defined 85-mm retroareolar mass. (**b**) Ultrasound shows multiple hypoechoic mass lesions which are ill-defined. (**c**) This is associated with increased dermal thickening and increased echogenicity of the intramammary fat mimicking inflammatory carcinoma. (**d**) Enlarged left axillary nodes are also present. Core biopsy of the mass and axillary node showed granulomatous mastitis and reactive axillary adenopathy

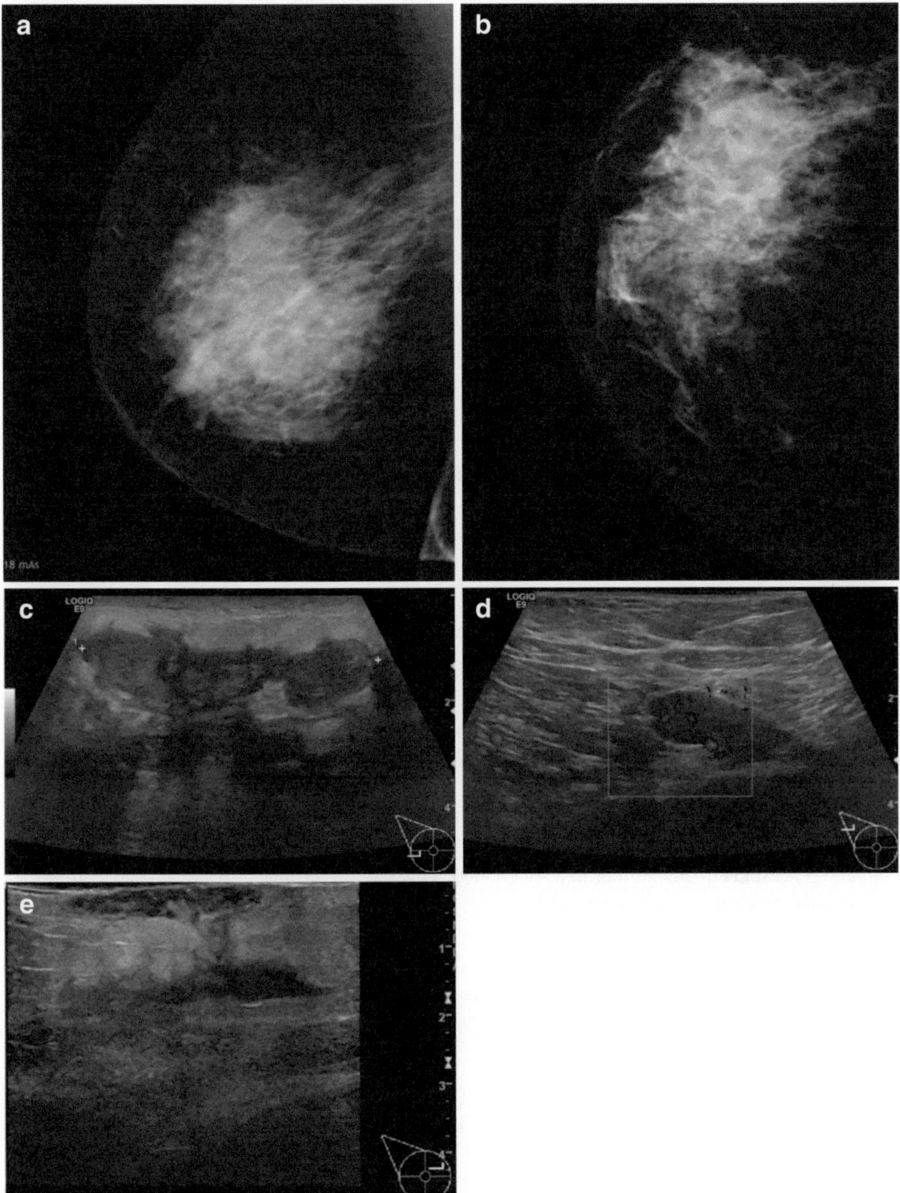

Fig. 3 (**a, b**) A 51-year-old woman with a 45-mm firm mass in the right breast with nipple retraction, peau d'orange, and suspicious adenopathy thought to be inflammatory carcinoma. Mammograms show an ill-defined 47-mm mass in the right breast. (**c**) Ultrasound shows a 55-mm ill-defined mass with surrounding inflammatory change and dermal thickening. (**d**) There are also abnormal right axillary nodes. (**e**) There was subsequent development of an inflammatory mass with a sinus tract extending into the skin. Core biopsy of the right breast and axilla shows granulomatous mastitis with negative screens for sarcoidosis and tuberculosis

4 Ultrasound

As with mammography, the sonographic appearances of IGM are varied. In early cases edema can be the only manifestation. US can demonstrate parenchymal heterogeneity and distortion [3] as well as ill-defined serpiginous hypoechoic areas which over time can become confluent to form masses. The most common finding on US is that of a hypoechoic irregular mass (Figs. 2 and 3) with peripheral hyperechogenicity. The mass often demonstrates tubular extensions [6] reflecting the propensity of IGM to interdigitate and insinuate between breast lobules rather than to engulf or destroy them [2] (Fig. 4). Posterior acoustic shadowing or enhancement is of little diagnostic relevance [2]. The pathological changes can occur in any quadrant of the breast but most commonly occurs in the retroareolar region (Fig. 5).

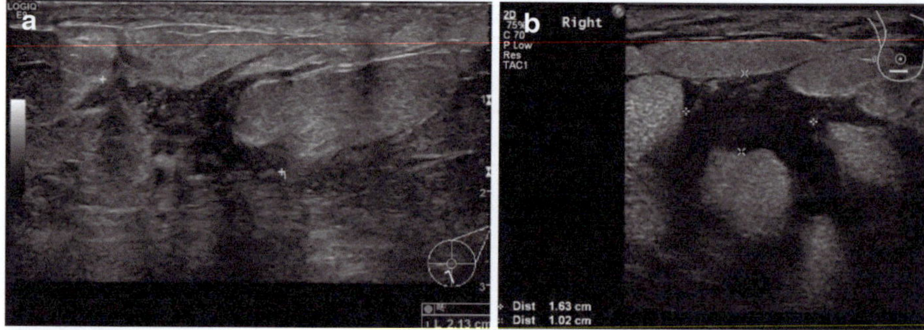

Fig. 4 Interdigitating extension of hypoechoic change between the fatty lobules on ultrasound. Hyperechoic change of the intramammary fatty lobules is also present. This appearance is nonspecific and represents diffuse inflammatory change. This can be present in IGM (**4a**) as well as lactational (**4b**) and non-lactational mastitis

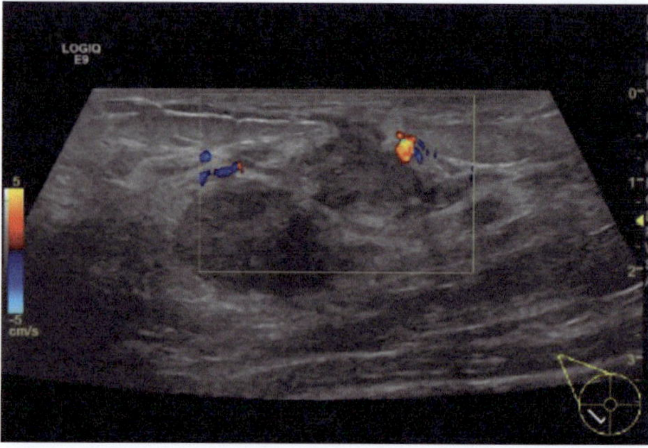

Fig. 5 A 43-year-old woman presenting with a right retroareolar mass with longstanding nipple inversion. Ultrasound-guided core biopsy showed granulomatous inflammation

The lesion and surrounding parenchyma are often edematous and can be hypervascular confirmed with Doppler imaging [5, 7]. Parenchymal heterogeneity [3], dermal thickening, and nipple retraction are common ancillary features (Fig. 2). In severe cases the patient can present with complex cystic collections and abscess formation which can be aspirated and a sample sent for microscopy, culture, and sensitivity as well as for cytology (Fig. 6). A sinus can develop, seen as an associated tract extending from the parenchymal hypoechoic inflammatory change to the skin surface (Fig. 7).

US can be helpful in the assessment of associated adenopathy (Figs. 2d and 3d). Enlarged lymph nodes can be present that demonstrate normal morphological appearances but with a thickened cortex in keeping with a reactive etiology.

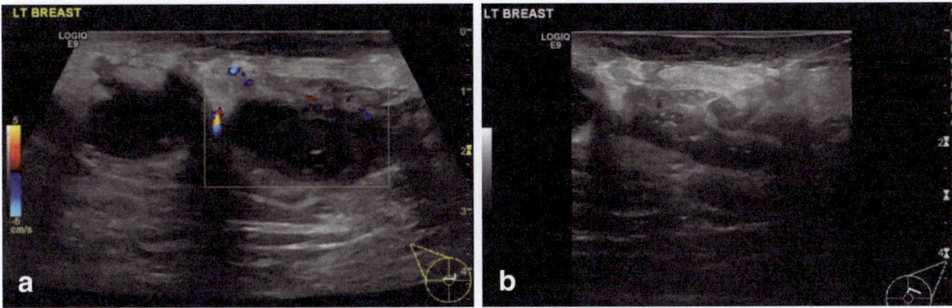

Fig. 6 (**a**) A 31-year-old woman with recurrent breast abscess. Ultrasound shows two collections with internal complex echoes with surrounding parenchymal inflammation with hypervascularity. (**b**) Ultrasound-guided aspiration

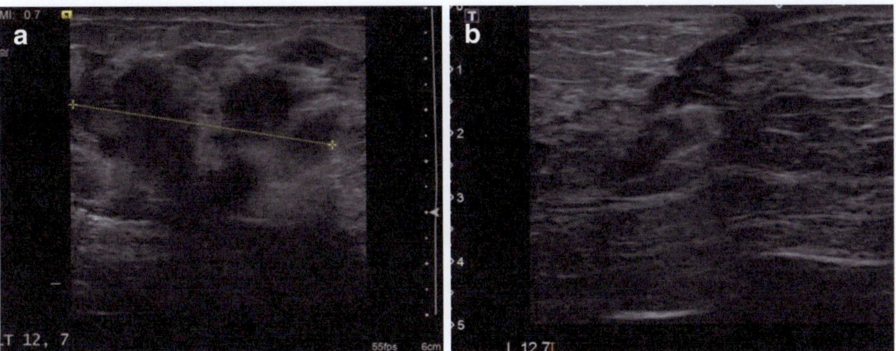

Fig. 7 (**a**) Sequelae of granulomatous mastitis. A 32-year-old woman presenting with painful diffuse lump in the left breast. (**b**) Subsequent development of a sinus tract 8 months later. There is an ill-defined hypervascular microlobulated mass in the 12:00 position of the left breast on ultrasound. Core biopsy confirmed granulomatous mastitis

5 Magnetic Resonance Imaging

Like other imaging modalities, MRI appearances of IGM can be variable and non-specific although MRI does appear to provide the best estimate of disease extent and contralateral breast involvement [8]. MRI is often utilized in the more challenging and refractory cases for monitoring disease progression and to assess response to treatment [2, 5]. IGM can be seen as irregular enhancing masses as well as asymmetric segmental non-mass enhancement. The largest case series by Yilmaz et al. [9] described heterogeneously enhancing masses as the dominant finding [10]. Diffuse non-mass enhancement is less commonly present [11]. IGM can also manifest as clustered well-circumscribed rounded lesions that are high signal on T2 and low signal on T1 with peripheral ring enhancement representing microabscess formation [5, 9, 10]. The majority of cases demonstrate a mixed enhancement pattern often with progressive wash-in and/or plateauing of the enhancement curve (Fig. 8) [12]. Regardless of the enhancement parametrics, the affected parenchyma is usually hyperenhancing compared with the normal breast tissue [8].

Accompanying perilesional edema, duct ectasia and periductal enhancement are recognized associations. Architectural distortion, sinus formation, and skin thickening are best visualized on T1 sequences. Oztekin et al. [12] found the majority (86%) of patients in a relatively small study of 29 patients to demonstrate a frank abscess; however, this is not a common finding in other centers.

Affected areas of the breast can demonstrate moderately restricted diffusion with consistently lower mean ADC values than the surrounding normal breast tissue [5, 8]; however, the use of restriction as a definitive diagnostic tool is of limited value in IGM [10].

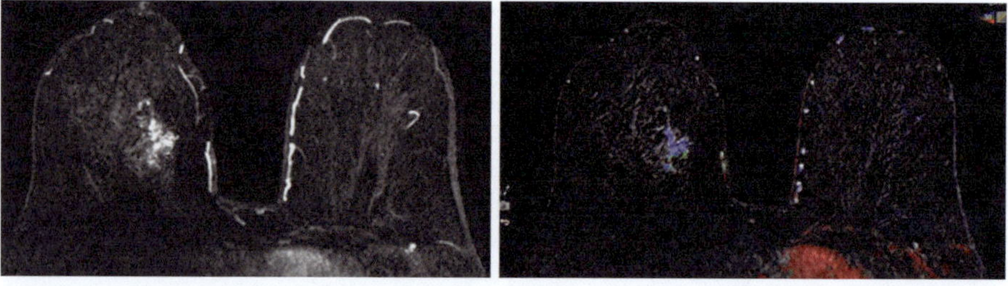

Fig. 8 A 54-year-old woman presenting with clinical suspicious 41-mm (US) breast mass in the upper inner quadrant of the right breast. Ultrasound-guided core biopsy showed benign histology (moderate chronic lymphoid infiltrate, no atypia or malignancy) felt to be discordant with the ill-defined type 1 non-mass enhancement on MRI. MRI-guided biopsy confirmed perilobular chronic mastitis

6   Computed Tomography

This modality is not a useful imaging tool in cases of IGM.

7   Other Conditions that Can Mimic IGM

7.1   *Infective Mastitis*

This is the most common cause of nonmalignant inflammatory breast disease in women of childbearing age and can be seen in both lactating and nonlactating women [2]. Imaging appearances of infective mastitis can be similar to IGM. Mammographic findings of both pathologies can be that of trabecular thickening and glandular asymmetry with parenchymal heterogeneity seen on US [2].

A spectrum of inflammatory change can be seen in both pathologies including subtle serpiginous pockets of fluid, complex coalescing fluid collections with mobile internal debris, or thick-walled, loculated formed abscesses, more likely to be seen in chronic or severe cases (Figs. 9, 10, 11 and 12). Patients who do not appear to respond to multiple courses of antibiotic therapy require investigation for infection caused by more atypical infections and to exclude other breast pathologies. By definition granulomatous mastitis should yield negative cultures [2].

Other forms of noninfective mastitis have similar imaging appearances (Figs. 13 and 14).

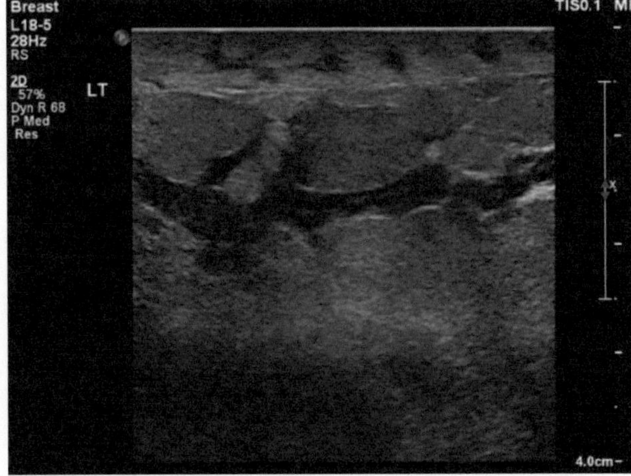

Fig. 9 A 41-year-old postpartum patient with left breast pain and erythema. Ultrasound confirms increased echogenicity with dermal and lymphatic thickening with no collection or abscess in keeping with mastitis

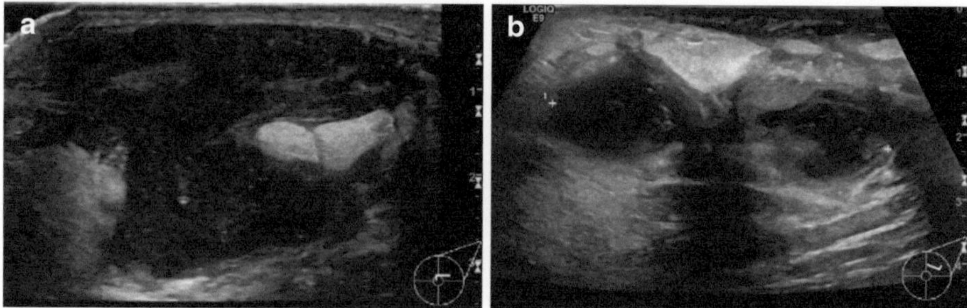

Fig. 10 (**a**) A 31-year-old breastfeeding patient presenting with a 4-week history of 41-mm complex lactational abscess. This was drained yielding heavy growth of *Staph. aureus* sensitive to flucloxacillin. (**b**) Improvement with follow-up scans and repeat percutaneous drainage

Fig. 11 A 33-year-old woman with right lactational mastitis showing interdigitating hypoechoic change between the fatty lobules against a background of increased echogenicity and dermal thickening

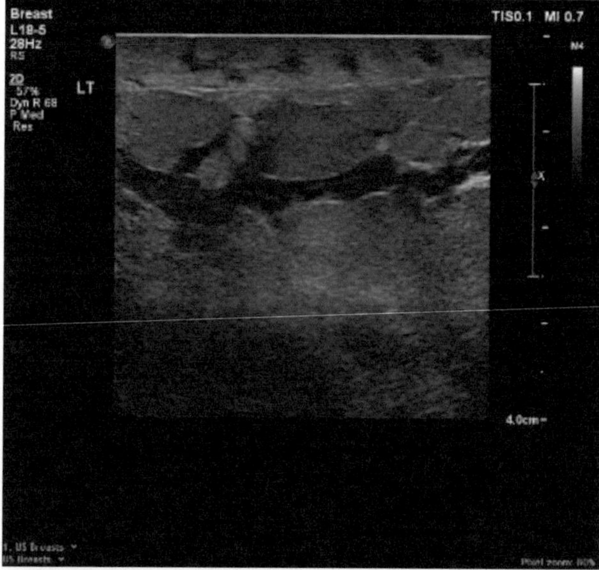

Fig. 12 A 26-year-old breastfeeding patient with a 2-week history of mastitis in the right breast. Ultrasound shows a large 70-mm complex collection confirmed to be an infected galactocele

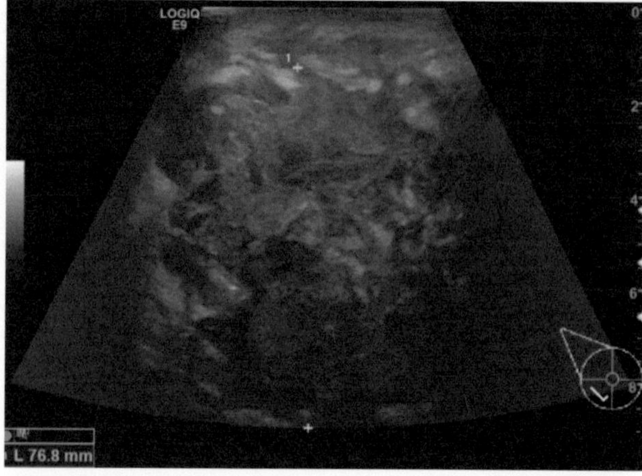

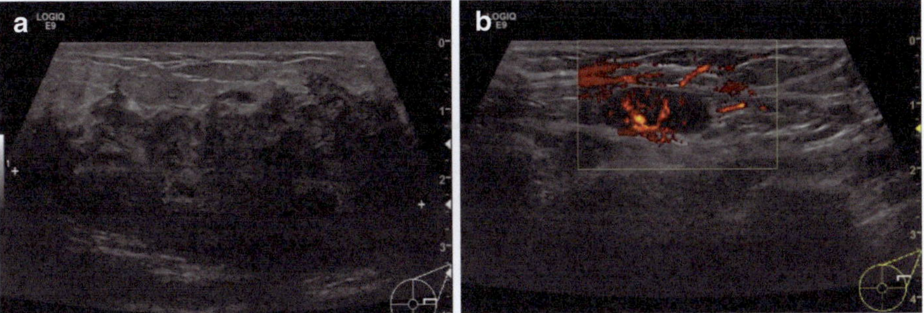

Fig. 13 (**a**) A 31-year-old woman presenting with a 5-day history of left breast swelling and pain. On ultrasound, there is a large 65-mm inflammatory mass occupying the lateral aspect of the left breast with no obvious collection. (**b**) Hypervascular enlarged nodes are also present. Core biopsy showed features in keeping with chronic mastitis with no granulomas

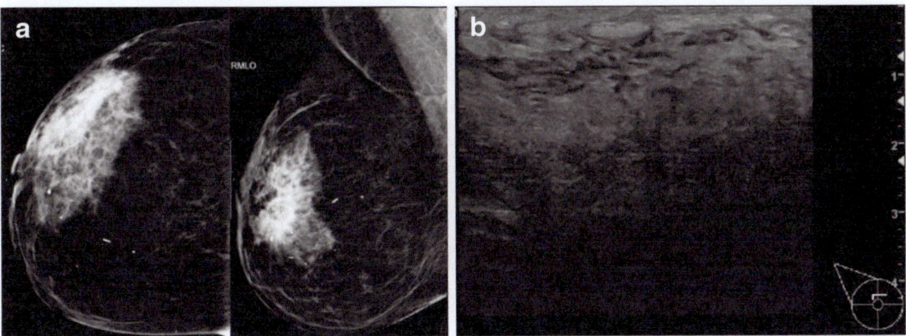

Fig. 14 (**a**) A 53-year-old woman presenting with 60-mm suspicious right retroareolar mass with right retroareolar asymmetry on mammography. (**b**) Diffuse inflammatory change centrally in the right breast on ultrasound. Core biopsy shows features in keeping with chronic mastitis. Subsequent follow-up confirmed complete clinical and imaging resolution

7.2 Periductal Mastitis

This is a form of mastitis occurring in nonlactating women and strongly associated with cigarette smoking. It most commonly affects women in their fourth decade but can affect all age groups and occasionally male patients [13]. The pathophysiology involves epithelial proliferation of the lactiferous ducts resulting in obstruction of secretions that can lead to infection often with *Staphylococcus aureus* and abscess formation. There is a propensity for infections to subsequently recur with mixed flora including anaerobic organisms that are more resistant to treatment. This can result in a more complex clinical course including fistulous tracts to the nipple areolar complex with a tendency for the infective changes to be centered on the periareolar region (Figs. 15 and 16) [13]. The radiological findings can be very similar to that of both IGM and inflammatory breast carcinoma. Periductal mastitis can been

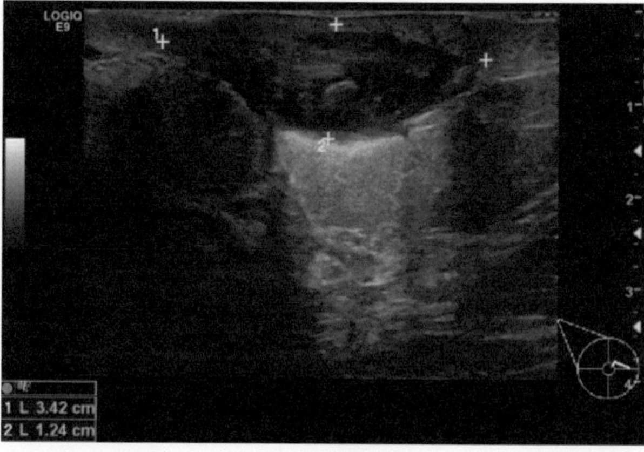

Fig. 15 A 36-year-old woman with recurrent right retroareolar collections in keeping with periductal mastitis

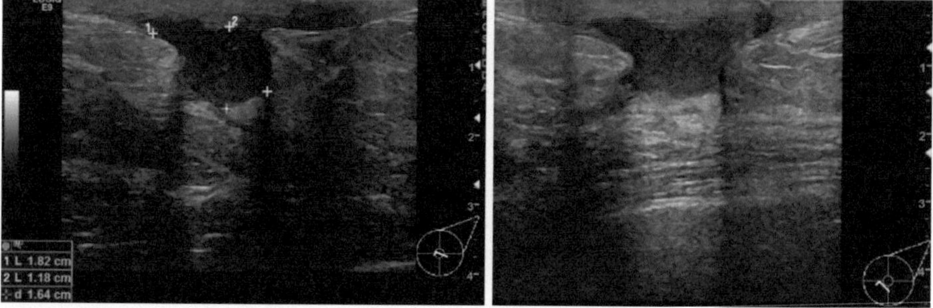

Fig. 16 A 41-year-old woman with recurrent left retroareolar collections. Periductal mastitis was confirmed on several biopsies

seen as a retroareolar opacity on mammography correlating with an ill-defined, mixed reflectivity collection on US. Reactive hyperemia can be present on US with surrounding parenchymal edema and dermal thickening. The sub areolar collection can be seen as a T2 hyperintense cystic mass on MRI which demonstrates peripheral enhancement on a postcontrast T1 fat-saturated subtracted sequence [13].

7.3 Tuberculous Mastitis

The prominent English surgeon Sir Astley Cooper [14] reported the first case of tuberculous mastitis in 1829 [15]. Multiparous and lactating women between the ages of 20 and 40 years are more frequently affected [15]; however, tuberculous mastitis is within the differential diagnosis of any patient presenting with diffuse inflammatory change within the breast, a painful mass, or abscess [16]. Both tuberculous mastitis and IGM can present with similar nonspecific radiological features; therefore, a clinical history of tuberculosis (TB) and/ or radiological manifestations of systemic or pulmonary TB can be helpful in differentiating between the two disease entities.

Breast tuberculosis has been divided into five types: nodular tuberculous mastitis, tuberculous mastitis obliterans, sclerosing tuberculous mastitis, disseminated tuberculous mastitis, and acute miliary tuberculous mastitis [15, 17].

Radiologically, there are three subtypes of tuberculous mastitis with distinguishing imaging features: nodular, diffuse, and sclerosing [18].

Mammographic findings can include diffuse trabecular thickening, areas of asymmetric focal density, or mass lesions which can be either solitary or multiple. The nodular form of tuberculosis can manifest as either a heterogenous ill-defined mass concerning for malignancy or a well-circumscribed benign-appearing lesion with similar imaging appearances to a fibroadenoma [15, 16]. Seo et al. [19] found that the most common imaging presentation in both TB and IGM was that of a mass which in some cases had suspicious radiological features mimicking malignancy [2]. In a study by Kilic et al. [20], 43.5% of breast tuberculosis cases were found to have been reported as BI-RADS 4/5 lesions.

As the name suggests, the diffuse form of the disease manifests as a more infiltrative parenchymal asymmetric density on mammography. The sclerosing subtype is more likely to occur in older women and the imaging appearances reflect the underlying pathological process involving extensive fibrosis. This is seen on mammography as a dense breast mass, often accompanied by nipple retraction and reduction in breast volume [15] (Fig. 17).

Sonographic features of both TB and IGM are similar to other granulomatous disorders of the breast as well as to malignancy. Parenchymal hyporeflectivity with surrounding inflammatory change, dermal thickening, solitary or multiple masses, and/or complex cystic collections are common findings of both entities. Communication can be seen between the masses in both TB and IGM as well as sinus tract formation extending to the skin surface [16]. The nodular subtype has similar US features to that seen on mammography presenting with a mass that can have either irregular or well-defined margins [15]. Confluent ill-defined masses can be seen in the diffuse form of tuberculous mastitis. Heterogeneous parenchyma with increased reflectivity but in the absence of a mass is a more common finding in the sclerosing subtype [15].

On MRI tuberculous mastitis tends to demonstrate a background of nonspecific parenchymal enhancement with edema and dermal thickening. More lesional ill-defined mass like areas of inflammatory involvement can be seen which demonstrate rapid contrast uptake and plateauing of the enhancement curve on T1-weighted imaging [15]. Abscess formation is typically hyperintense on T2 with peripheral ring enhancement and central necrosis. Sinus formation and fistulation are both well visualized on MRI and fistulous extension into deeper tissues can also be more clearly depicted, particularly on the T1 sequence [15].

Ancillary findings of tuberculous mastitis include coarse calcifications, skin thickening, duct ectasia, nipple retraction, and lymphadenopathy [16]. The presence of calcified axillary lymph nodes can help to differentiate TB from IGM or malignancy [18].

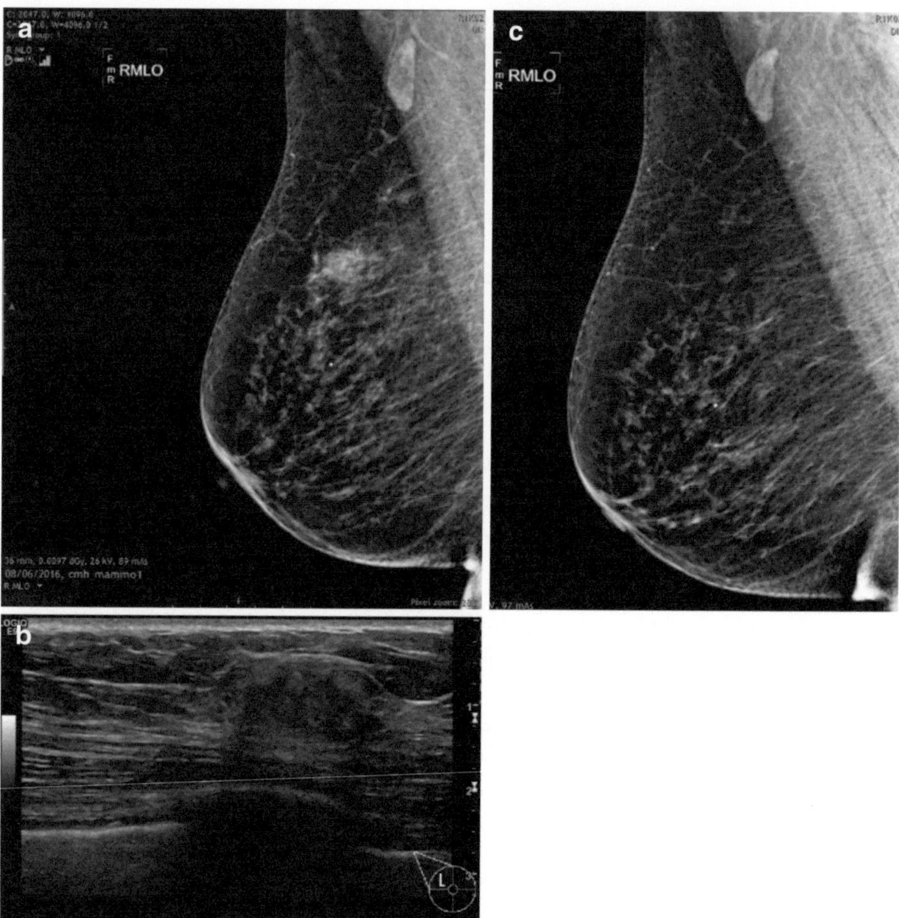

Fig. 17 (a) A 57-year-old woman with previous left breast cancer. Mammograms show a new ill-defined mass in the right upper outer quadrant. (b) A 20-mm ill-defined mass on ultrasound thought to be a new malignant mass. Core biopsy showed changes in keeping with granulomatous mastitis. Further core biopsies were performed for microbiological cultures and stainings, TB cultures, and 16S rDNA PCR test to diagnose TB. (c) Right mammogram showing full resolution of the mass a year later following antituberculous treatment

The axillary lymph nodes in TB are likely to be enlarged and can demonstrate cortical thickening; however, the margin of the involved nodes tend to be smooth and regular with a normal fatty hilum and preservation of the nodal architecture. These appearances are therefore more likely to reflect a benign or reactive/inflammatory etiology rather than a malignant process. In particularly severe cases of TB mastitis, a confluent nodal mass can form in the axilla which can be centrally necrotic and which has the potential to form a sinus tract to the overlying skin surface.

Diagnosis is usually confirmed by tissue sampling of the affected breast detecting acid-fast bacilli on Ziehl-Neelsen staining or cultures or performing a 16S rDNA PCR test.

7.4 Sarcoidosis

Sarcoidosis is a disease of the immune system which can affect any organ or system [2]. Breast involvement is rare, occurring in less than 1% of patients with systemic sarcoidosis [21]. Sarcoidosis most commonly affects young females and can present as a firm, hard breast mass in the context of involvement of other organs and in the presence of a raised angiotensin-converting enzyme [21]. Unilateral or bilateral, irregular or spiculate masses are the most common finding on mammography [22]. Ill-defined hypoechoic masses are the most common US presentation although small well-defined masses have also been described. Interestingly, calcifications are typically not seen [21, 22]. Irregular heterogeneously enhancing masses can be seen on MRI demonstrating type 2/3 enhancement parametrics.

7.5 Malignancy

As previously described, the most common clinical symptoms of IGM include an asymmetrically enlarged breast, erythema, edema, unilateral palpable breast mass, nipple retraction, and axillary lymphadenopathy. These signs and symptoms are also frequent presenting features of breast malignancy, in particular inflammatory breast carcinoma which is defined as a histological diagnosis of malignancy in the context of a clinically apparent inflammatory process. The similarities between these two entities mean that they are often clinically and radiologically indistinguishable (Figs. 18 and 19).

Extensive dermal edema and trabecular thickening seen on both mammography and sonography can occur in both inflammatory breast cancer and IGM, but are seen less commonly in the latter [2]. Breast mass, asymmetric density, and distortion are imaging findings common to both disease processes and are less discriminatory [2]. The presence of an abscess and/or sinus tract can be a useful diagnostic feature favoring an underlying diagnosis of IGM rather than malignancy.

As with other imaging modalities, similar MRI features can be present in both IGM and malignancy, and therefore, MRI cannot be used to confidently distinguish between these two pathologies. Both disease processes can manifest as heterogeneously enhancing masses on dynamic T1 fat-saturated sequences; however, a malignant pathology is more likely to demonstrate early wash-in of contrast with rapid washout compared with plateauing of the enhancement curve seen with

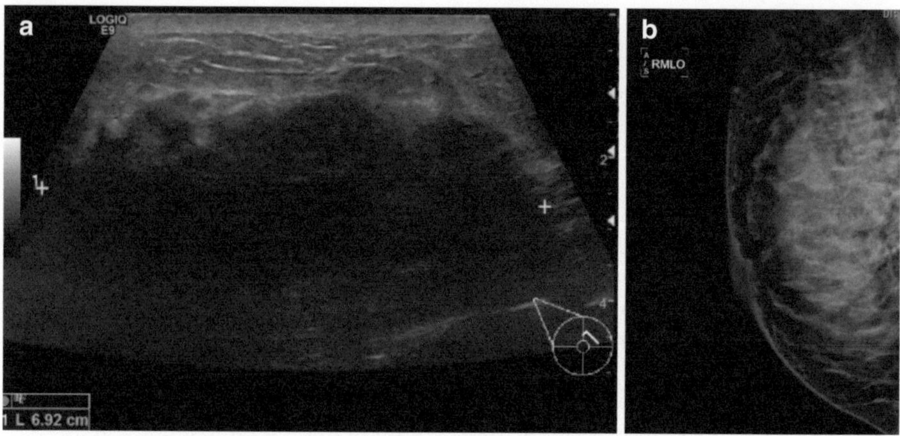

Fig. 18 (**a**) A 32-year-old woman who is 12 weeks' pregnant presenting with inflammatory change in her right breast thought to be an abscess. Core biopsy showed node-positive grade 2 invasive ductal carcinoma ER4/8 PR2/8 HER2 positive. (**b**) Mammography shows diffuse edematous change and skin thickening in keeping with inflammatory breast cancer

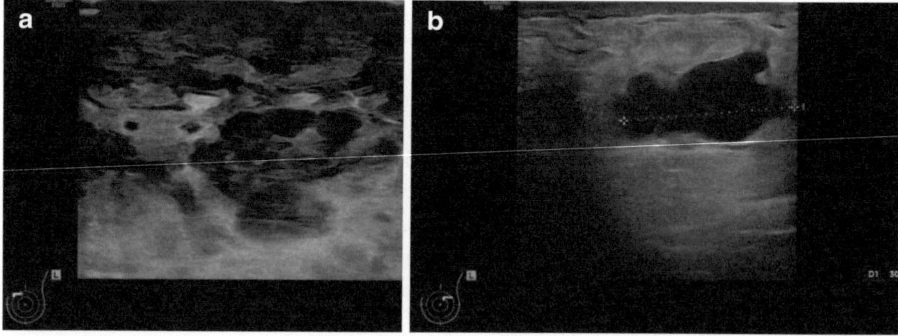

Fig. 19 An 86-year-old woman presenting with peau d'orange and enlarged left breast thought to represent a locally advanced breast cancer. Ultrasound shows (**a**) dermal and subcutaneous nodules and inflammatory change as well as (**b**) multiple lobulated masses. Core biopsy shows this to be lymphoma

IGM. Asymmetric and/or segmental non-mass enhancement is another common MRI finding of both pathologies [2]. The mass lesions seen in IGM are commonly rim enhancing with a smooth margin. This observation was supported by Poyraz et al. [23] whose study confirmed that the mass lesions seen in IGM are more likely to be well defined and rounded with rim enhancement rather than the ill-defined, irregular masses most likely to be seen in malignancy.

If breast malignancy is associated with nodal involvement, the lymph nodes can have pathological imaging appearance. Such features include nodal enlargement, rounded morphology, and loss of the normal nodal architecture with cortical effacement. The nodes in IGM are characteristically enlarged; however, they are more likely to exhibit a normal morphology with preservation of the fatty hilum.

7.6 *Diabetic Mastopathy*

Diabetic mastopathy is a relatively uncommon benign condition occurring in patients with a long history of insulin-dependent diabetes mellitus characteristically in premenopausal women approximately 20 years after the onset of their diabetes [13, 22]. Such patients tend to present clinically with large, firm, non-tender solitary, or multiple breast masses that can sometimes be bilateral. Both the clinical findings and imaging appearances of diabetic mastopathy are often concerning for and indistinguishable from malignancy (Fig. 20).

Both IGM and diabetic mastopathy can present with irregular masses or heterogeneous asymmetric densities on mammography. Diabetic mastopathy is more commonly bilateral when compared with either IGM or breast malignancy. Hypoechoic masses or ill-defined areas of hyporeflectivity can be seen on US, often with significant posterior acoustic shadowing [13]. There is limited published data on MRI findings of diabetic mastopathy; however, the most frequently encountered appearances are seen to be that of patchy parenchymal enhancement [24]. Given the nonspecific imaging characteristics, tissue sampling is warranted to distinguish between the breast pathologies.

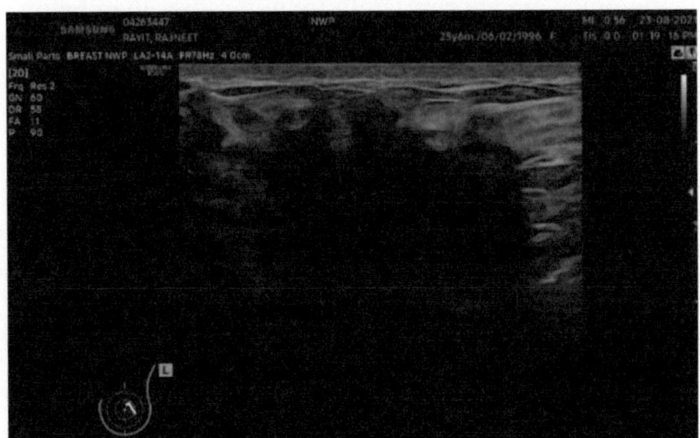

Fig. 20 A 35-year-old insulin-dependent diabetic patient with painful inflamed lump in the left breast. Ultrasound shows an ill-defined heterogeneous lobulated hypoechoic mass. Core biopsy confirmed diabetic mastopathy

7.7 Mastitis in Other Autoimmune Conditions

Autoimmune mastitis has only relatively recently been described in the literature with increasing numbers of case reports suggesting that this condition has previously been underdiagnosed. Many autoimmune conditions with multisystem involvement also have the potential to manifest as breast pathology. Autoimmune mastitis includes a wide range of disease entities including Wegener's granulomatosis, IgG4 disease, Sjogren's disease, Crohn's disease, systemic lupus erythematosus, thyroiditis, eosinophilic mastitis, and amyloidosis [25]. The clinical presentation of autoimmune mastitis can be varied ranging from minimal symptoms to recurrent episodes of severe inflammation and discharging abscess. Dermal involvement, nipple retraction, and lymphadenopathy have also been reported [25]. Radiological appearances are often similar to IGM and can include a focal mass or can present as a more diffuse nonspecific imaging finding.

8 Conclusion

In summary, IGM is a rare benign inflammatory condition of the breast characterized by noncaseating granulomatous formation without an attributable cause. IGM commonly occurs in premenopausal women and has a spectrum of nondiscriminatory imaging appearances mimicking both benign and malignant conditions resulting in a prolonged and tortuous diagnostic path. The diagnosis of IGM is one of exclusion and can therefore only be established after imaging-guided tissue sampling has eliminated other causes of inflammatory breast diseases (Fig. 21). Correlation with clinical history and examination findings as well as MDT discussion are vital in establishing the correct diagnosis and treatment plan. This helps to ensure that cases of malignancy are diagnosed in a timely fashion and that benign pathologies are appropriately treated rather than being subjected to radical surgical intervention.

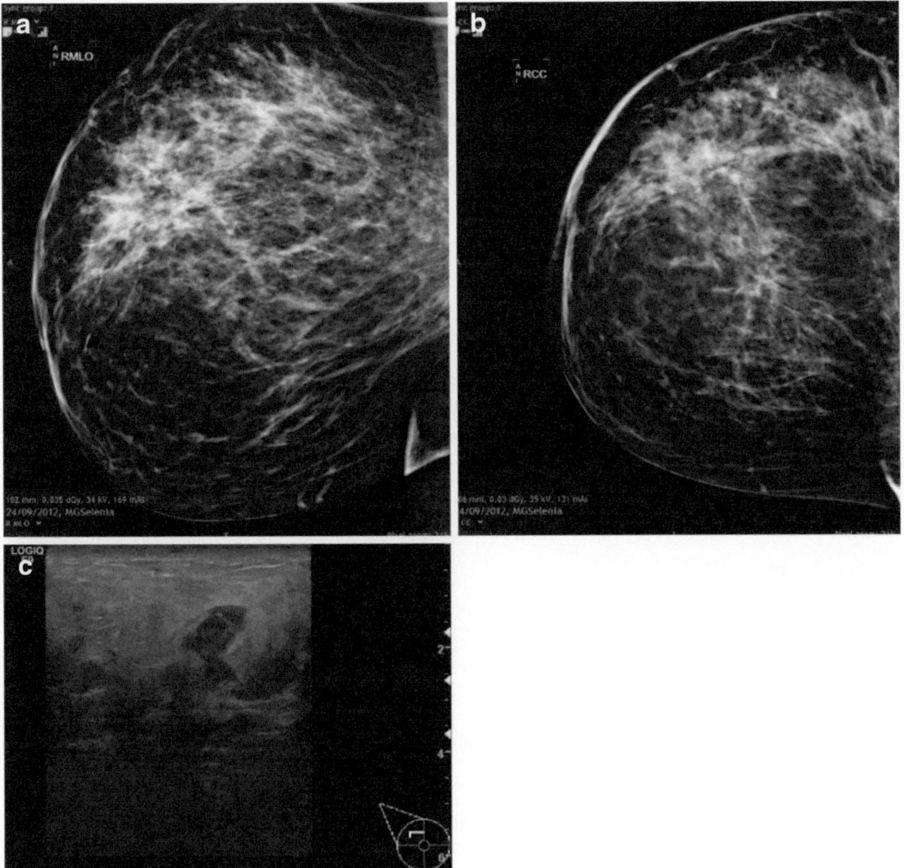

Fig. 21 (**a**, **b**) A 38-year-old woman presented with diffusely tense, red, and swollen right breast. Mammograms show diffuse thickening of the dermis associated with increased trabecular pattern and asymmetrical density in the superior and lateral aspect of the right breast. (**c**) Ultrasound shows right upper outer quadrant diffuse edema of the dermis and intramammary fat associated with thickening of Cooper's ligaments associated with multiple hypoechoic lesions. Core biopsy confirms granulomatous mastitis. (**d**, **e**) Mammograms later show normal right breast

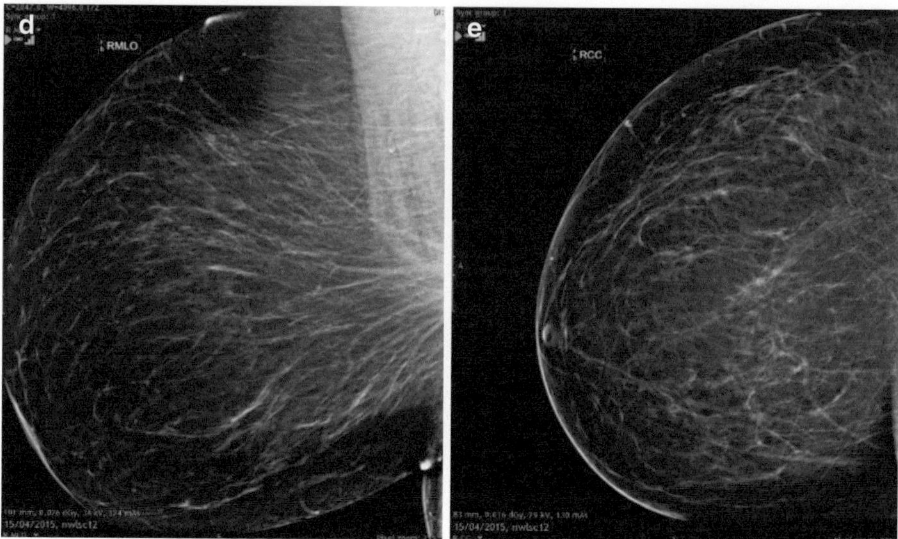

Fig. 21 (continued)

References

1. Kessler E, Wolloch Y. Granulomatous mastitis: a lesion clinically simulating carcinoma. Am J Clin Pathol. 1972;58:642–6. https://doi.org/10.1093/ajcp/58.6.642.
2. Pluguez-Turull CW, Nanyes JE, Quintero CJ, Alizai H, Mais DD, Kist KA, et al. Idiopathic granulomatous mastitis: manifestations at multimodality imaging and pitfalls. Radiographics. 2018;38(2):330–56. https://doi.org/10.1148/rg.2018170095.
3. Gurleyik G, Aktekin A, Aker F, Karagulle H, Saglam A. Medical and surgical treatment of idiopathic granulomatous lobular mastitis: a benign inflammatory disease mimicking invasive carcinoma. J Breast Cancer. 2012;15:119–23. https://doi.org/10.4048/jbc.2012.15.1.119.
4. Tardivon AA, Viala J, Corvellec Rudelli A, Guinebretiere JM, Vanel D. Mammographic patterns of inflammatory breast carcinoma: a retrospective study of 92 cases. Eur J Radiol. 1997;24:124–30. https://doi.org/10.1016/s0720-048x(96)01137-0.
5. Fazzio RT, Shah SS, Sandhu NP, Glazebrook KN. Idiopathic granulomatous mastitis: imaging update and review. Insights Imaging. 2016;7:531–9. https://doi.org/10.1007/s13244-016-0499-0.
6. Hovanessian Larsen LJ, Peyvandi B, Klipfel N, Grant E, Iyengar G. Granulomatous lobular mastitis: imaging, diagnosis, and treatment. AJR Am J Roentgenol. 2009;193:574–81. https://doi.org/10.2214/AJR.08.1528.
7. Handa P, Leibman AJ, Sun D, Abadi M, Goldberg A. Granulomatous mastitis: changing clinical and imaging features with image-guided biopsy correlation. Eur Radiol. 2014;24:2404–11. https://doi.org/10.1007/s00330-014-3273-z.
8. Manogna P, Dev B, Joseph LD, Ramakrishnan R. Idiopathic granulomatous mastitis-our experience. Egypt J Radiol Nucl Med. 2020;51:15. https://doi.org/10.1186/s43055-019-0126-4.
9. Yilmaz R, Demir AA, Kaplan A, Sahin D, Ozkurt E, Dursun M, et al. Magnetic resonance imaging features of idiopathic granulomatous mastitis: is there any contribution of diffusion-weighted imaging in the differential diagnosis? Radiol Med. 2016;121:857–66. https://doi.org/10.1007/s11547-016-0666-x.

10. Matich A, Sud S, Buxi TBS, Dogra V. Idiopathic granulomatous mastitis and its mimics on magnetic resonance imaging: a pictorial review of cases from India. J Clin Imaging Sci. 2020;10:53. https://doi.org/10.25259/JCIS_112_2019.

11. Dursun M, Yilmaz S, Yahyayev A, Salmaslioglu A, Yavuz E, Igci A, et al. Multimodality imaging features of idiopathic granulomatous mastitis: outcome of 12 years of experience. Radiol Med. 2012;117:529–38. https://doi.org/10.1007/s11547-011-0733-2.

12. Oztekin PS, Durhan G, Nercis Kosar P, Erel S, Hucumenoglu S. Imaging findings in patients with granulomatous mastitis. Iran J Radiol. 2016;13:e33900. https://doi.org/10.5812/iranjradiol.33900.

13. Leong PW, Chotai NC, Kulkarni S. Imaging features of inflammatory breast disorders: a pictorial essay. Korean J Radiol. 2018;19:5–14. https://doi.org/10.3348/kjr.2018.19.1.5.

14. Cooper A. Illustrations of the diseases of the breast. London: Longman CA, Rees O. Brown and Green; 1829.

15. Baykan AH, Sayiner HS, Inan I, Aydin E, Erturk SM. Primary breast tuberculosis: imaging findings of a rare disease. Insights Imaging. 2021;12:19. https://doi.org/10.1186/s13244-021-00961-3.

16. Farrokh D, Alamdaran A, Feyzi Laeen A, Fallah Rastegar Y, Abbasi B. Tuberculous mastitis: a review of 32 cases. Int J Infect Dis. 2019;87:135–42. https://doi.org/10.1016/j.ijid.2019.08.013.

17. Longman CF, Campion T, Butler B, Suaris TD, Khanam A, Kunst H, et al. Imaging features and diagnosis of tuberculosis of the breast. Clin Radiol. 2017;72:217–22. https://doi.org/10.1016/j.crad.2016.11.023.

18. Sakr AA, Fawzy RK, Fadaly G, Baky MA. Mammographic and sonographic features of tuberculous mastitis. Eur J Radiol. 2004;51:54–60. https://doi.org/10.1016/S0720-048X(03)00230-4.

19. Seo HR, Na KY, Yim HE, Kim TH, Kang DK, Oh KK, et al. Differential diagnosis in idiopathic granulomatous mastitis and tuberculous mastitis. J Breast Cancer. 2012;15:111–8. https://doi.org/10.4048/jbc.2012.15.1.111.

20. Kilic MO, Sağlam C, Ağca FD, Terzioğlu SG. Clinical, diagnostic and therapeutic management of patients with breast tuberculosis: analysis of 46 cases. Kaohsiung J Med Sci. 2016;32:27–31. https://doi.org/10.1016/j.kjms.2015.12.005.

21. Illman JE, Terra SB, Clapp AJ, Hunt KN, Fazzio RT, Shah SS, et al. Granulomatous diseases of the breast and axilla: radiological findings with pathological correlation. Insights Imaging. 2018;9:59–71. https://doi.org/10.1007/s13244-017-0587-9.

22. Sabaté JM, Clotet M, Gómez A, De Las HP, Torrubia S, Salinas T. Radiologic evaluation of uncommon inflammatory and reactive breast disorders. Radiographics. 2005;25:411–24. https://doi.org/10.1148/rg.252045077.

23. Poyraz N, Emlik GD, Batur A, Gundes E, Keskin S. Magnetic resonance imaging features of idiopathic granulomatous mastitis: a retrospective analysis. Iran J Radiol. 2016;13:e20873. https://doi.org/10.5812/iranjradiol.20873.

24. Wong KT, Tse GM, Yang WT. Ultrasound and MR imaging of diabetic mastopathy. Clin Radiol. 2002;57:730–5. https://doi.org/10.1053/crad.2002.0936.

25. Goulabchand R, Hafidi A, Van de Perre P, Millet I, Maria ATJ, Morel J, et al. Mastitis in autoimmune diseases: review of the literature, diagnostic pathway, and pathophysiological key players. J Clin Med. 2020;9:958. https://doi.org/10.3390/jcm9040958.

Pathology of Idiopathic Granulomatous Mastitis

Esra Yilmaz ⓘ

Firstly, Milward and Gough [1] reported a patient with granulomatous lesions in the breast, which was admitted with cancer-like clinical findings in the breast. In 1972, Kessler and Wolloch described this entity, and then Cohen [2] detailed the pathology of this entity. Until today, the criteria used in the diagnosis of IGM have not been changed much from the criteria defined by Kessler and Wolloch [3].

Although the pathological definitions are known, the diagnosis of IGM is one of exclusion usually. The causes of granulomatous inflammation in the breast are shown in Table 1.

E. Yilmaz (✉)
Department of Pathology, Saglik Bilimleri University, Hamidiye Faculty of Medicine, Ministry of Health, Konya City Hospital, Konya, Türkiye

Table 1 Causes of granulomatous inflammation in the breast

Causes
Infectious
Mycobacterium tuberculosis
Blastomycosis
Cryptococcosis
Histoplasmosis
Actinomycosis
Filarial infection
Corynebacterium
Autoimmune
Wegener granulomatosis
Giant cell arteritis
Foreign body reaction
Duct ectasis
Plasma cell mastitis
Subareolar granuloma
Periductal mastitis
Diabetes mellitus
Sarcoidosis
Fat necrosis
Idiopathic

1 Fine-Needle Aspiration Cytology

The diagnosis of IGM by fine-needle aspiration cytology (FNAC) is controversial because of overlapping features with other etiologies especially tuberculosis. Specific features for IGM are absent [4]. For the diagnosis of IGM, all other known causes of granulomatous inflammation must be excluded [5]. Whilst some studies in the literature support the useful role of FNAC, others mention that different causes of granulomatous inflammation cannot be differentiated exactly by FNAC [6, 7]. Even so, FNAC is still a notable alternative because of its availability and ease of use. Additionally, FNAC may help in differentiating malignancy and inflammation [6].

Cytologically epithelioid cell granulomas (Figs. 1, 2, 3, 4 and 5), single epithelioid cells, and multinucleated giant cells of foreign body and/or Langhans type are common findings of IGM [7–12]. Epithelioid cell granulomas cannot be demonstrated in all cases depending on, technically, undersampling [7, 8]. Caseous necrosis characterized by ground-glass eosinophilic material is also absent [5, 7, 8, 10, 11]. Necrosis associated with neutrophilic inflammation may be seen [8]. Inflammatory cells commonly consist of neutrophils (Figs. 6, 7, 8, 9 and 10) [7–9]. Lymphocytes, plasma cells, and scanty eosinophils can be seen in variable numbers [5, 7–13].

Fig. 1 Granulomas composed of epithelioid cells (HE × 100)

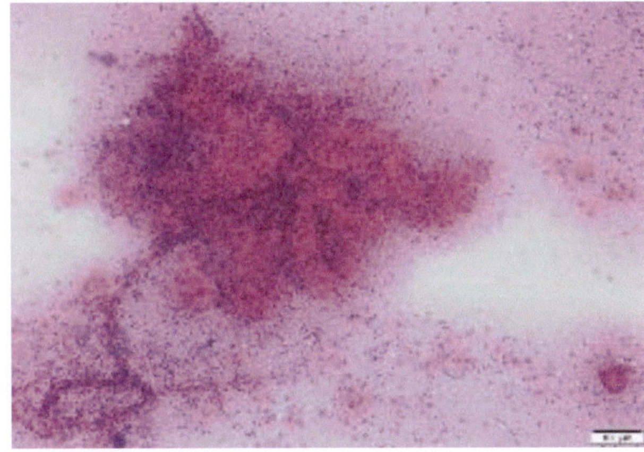

Fig. 2 Granulomas composed of epithelioid cells (PAP × 100)

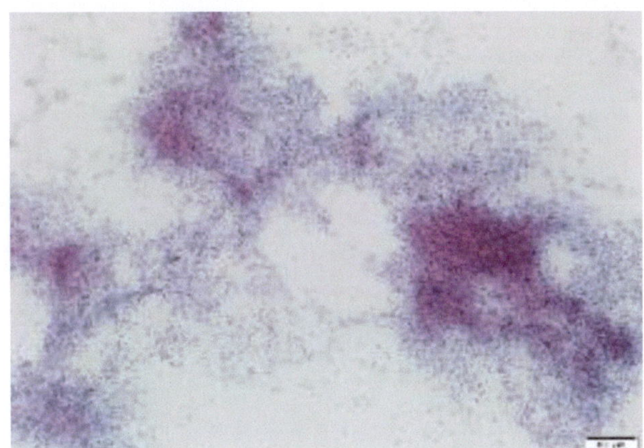

Fig. 3 Granulomas composed of epithelioid cells (PAP × 200)

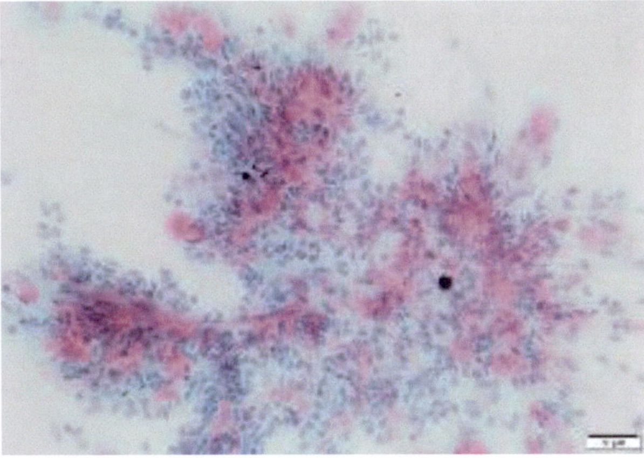

                                          E. Yilmaz

Fig. 4 Granulomas composed of epithelioid cells (HE × 200)

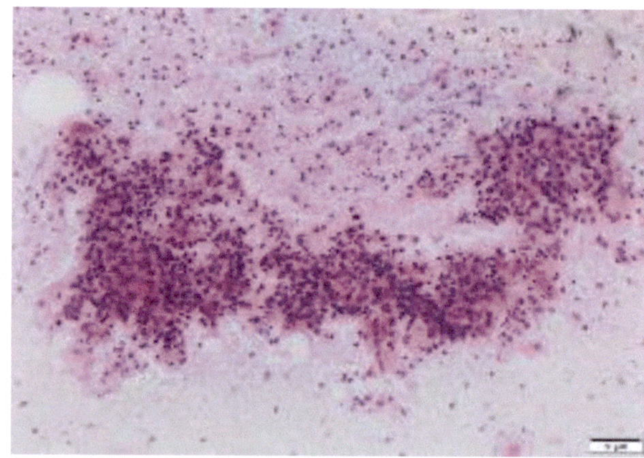

Fig. 5 Granulomas composed of epithelioid cells (HE × 400)

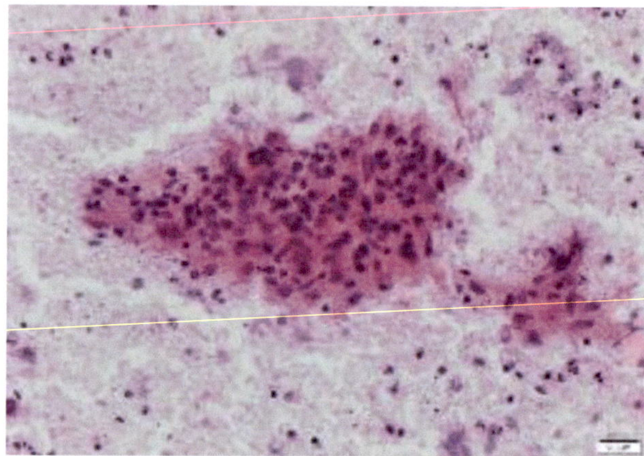

Fig. 6 Epithelioid cell granuloma with neutrophilic inflammation (HE × 200)

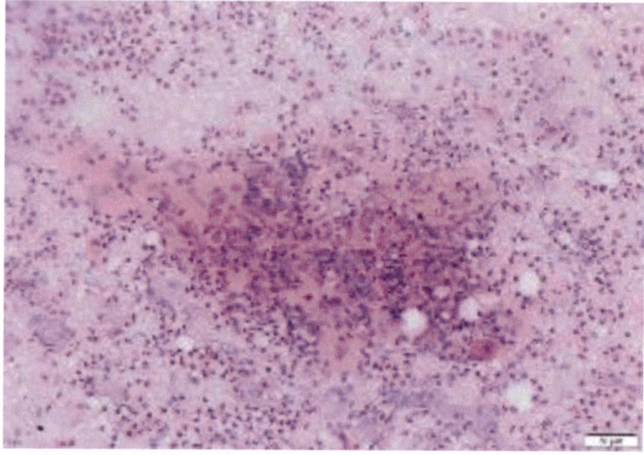

Fig. 7 Multinucleated giant cells, single epithelioid cells, and inflammatory cells commonly consist of neutrophils (HE × 200)

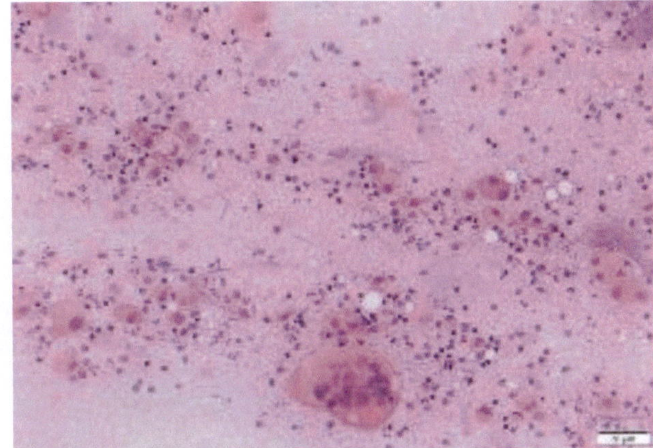

Fig. 8 Multinucleated giant cells, single epithelioid cells, and inflammatory cells commonly consist of neutrophils (HE × 400)

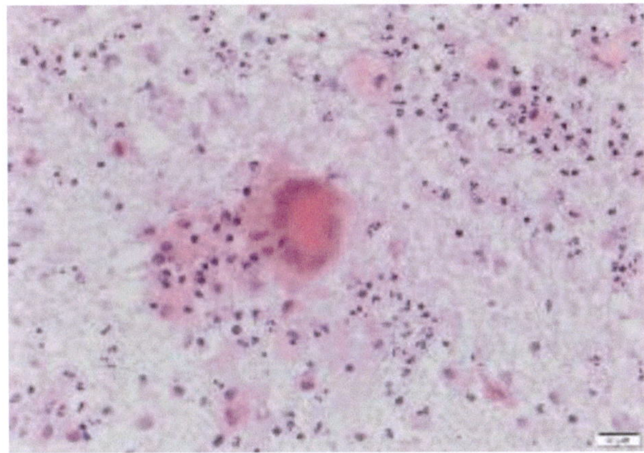

Fig. 9 Multinucleated giant cells, single epithelioid cells, and inflammatory cells commonly consist of neutrophils (HE × 200)

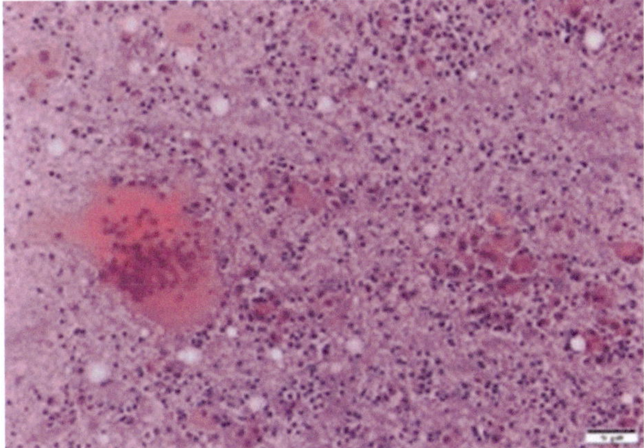

Fig. 10 Multinucleated giant cells, single epithelioid cells, and inflammatory cells commonly consist of neutrophils (HE × 400)

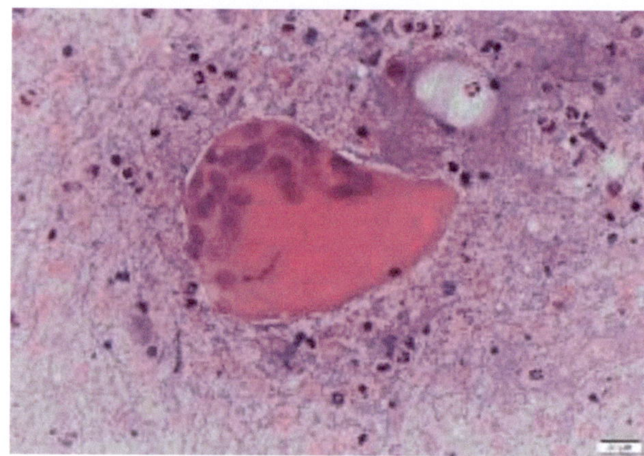

2 Gross Pathology

Macroscopic specimens typically consist of greyish-white to tan-colored cut surface with a faintly nodular architecture. In some cases, small foci of abscess formation can be seen [14, 15].

3 Histopathology

The major histopathologic change in IGM is non-necrotizing granulomatous inflammation centered in breast lobules with or without intralobular microabscess formation [16, 17]. Granulomas (Figs. 11, 12, 13, 14, 15, 16 and 17) include epithelioid histiocytes and multinucleated giant cells (Fig. 18, 19 and 20) with varying numbers of lymphocytes, plasma cells, neutrophils, and eosinophils (Figs. 21, 22 and 23) [16, 18, 19]. As a result of inflammatory progression, confluent granulomas, fat necrosis, abscess formation, and fibrosis can damage lobular architecture [14, 15]. The microcystic spaces seen in the center of abscesses do not contain foreign material or secretion (Figs. 24, 25, 26, 27 and 28) [14, 15]. Ductal or lobular epithelial squamous metaplasia is an unusual finding in IGM [14, 15].

Fig. 11 Non-necrotizing granulomatous inflammation. Granulomas composed of epithelioid histiocytes, multinucleated giant cells, and varying numbers of lymphocytes, plasma cells, neutrophils, and eosinophils (HE × 200)

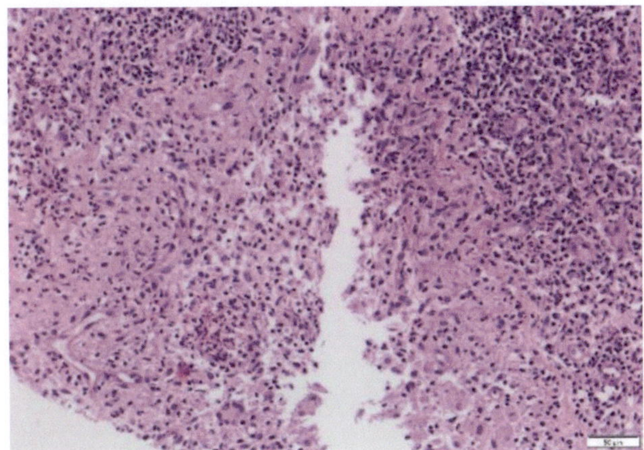

Fig. 12 Non-necrotizing granulomatous inflammation. Granulomas composed of epithelioid histiocytes, multinucleated giant cells, and varying numbers of lymphocytes, plasma cells, neutrophils, and eosinophils (HE × 200)

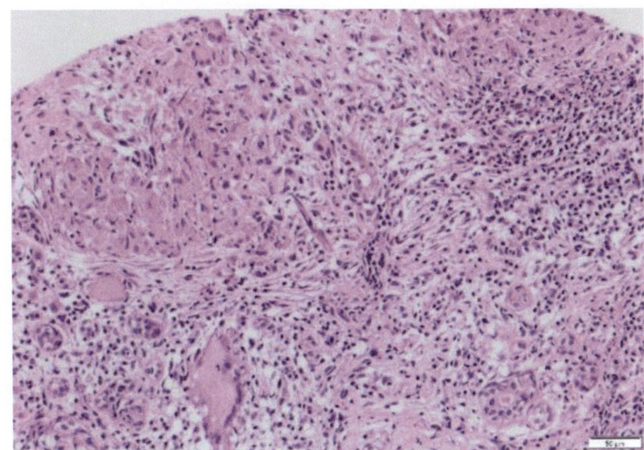

Fig. 13 Non-necrotizing granulomatous inflammation. Granulomas composed of epithelioid histiocytes, multinucleated giant cells, and varying numbers of lymphocytes, plasma cells, neutrophils, and eosinophils (HE × 200)

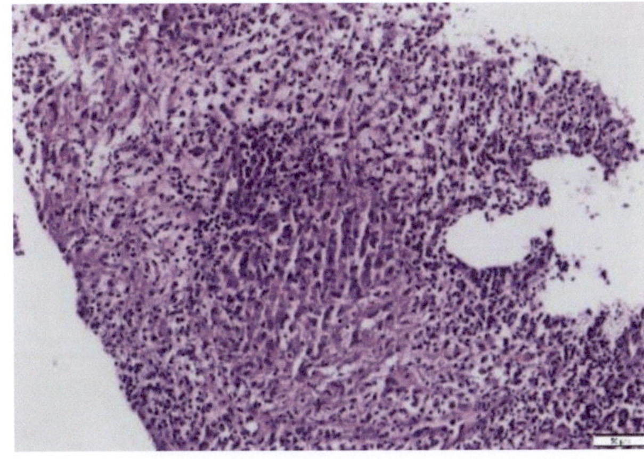

Fig. 14 Non-necrotizing granulomatous inflammation. Granulomas composed of epithelioid histiocytes, multinucleated giant cells, and varying numbers of lymphocytes, plasma cells, neutrophils, and eosinophils (HE × 200)

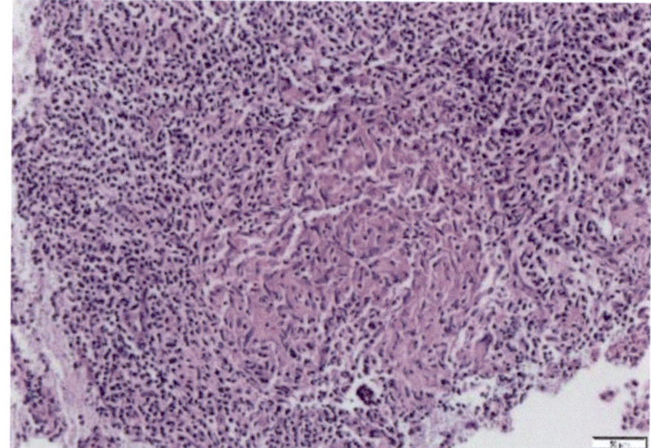

Fig. 15 Non-necrotizing granulomatous inflammation. Granulomas composed of epithelioid histiocytes, multinucleated giant cells, and varying numbers of lymphocytes, plasma cells, neutrophils, and eosinophils (HE × 200)

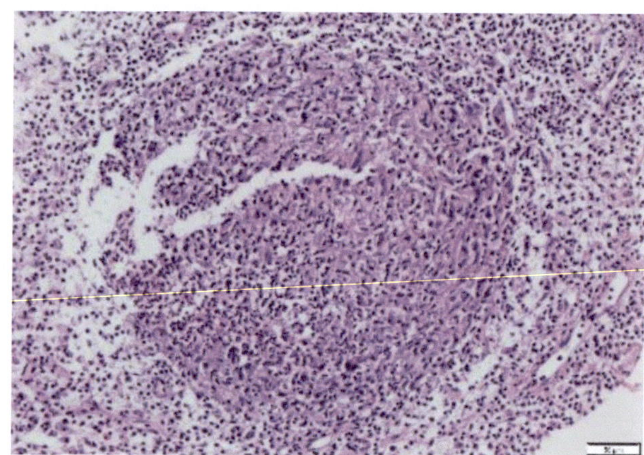

Fig. 16 Non-necrotizing granulomatous inflammation. Granulomas composed of epithelioid histiocytes, multinucleated giant cells, and varying numbers of lymphocytes, plasma cells, neutrophils, and eosinophils (HE × 400)

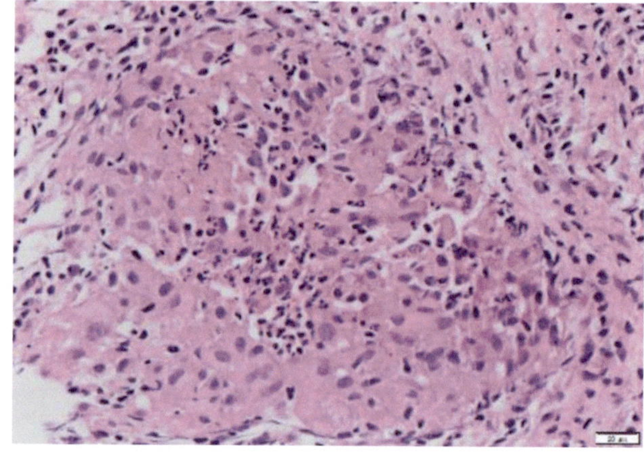

Fig. 17 Non-necrotizing granulomatous inflammation. Granulomas composed of epithelioid histiocytes, multinucleated giant cells, and varying numbers of lymphocytes, plasma cells, neutrophils, and eosinophils (HE × 400)

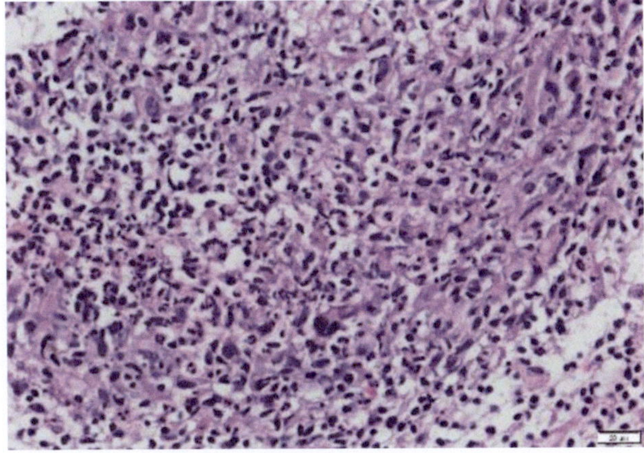

Fig. 18 Langhans-type multinucleated giant cells in granulomatous inflammation (HE × 400)

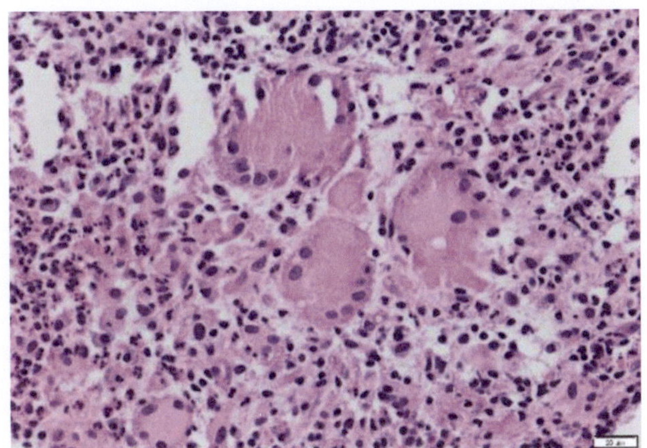

Fig. 19 Langhans-type multinucleated giant cells in granulomatous inflammation (HE × 400)

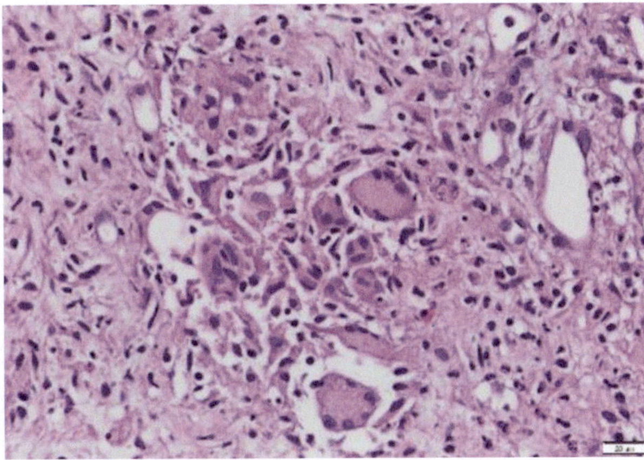

E. Yilmaz

Fig. 20 Langhans-type multinucleated giant cells in granulomatous inflammation (HE × 400)

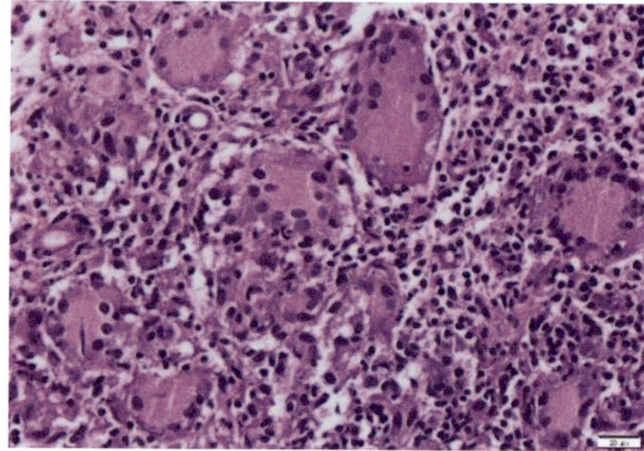

Fig. 21 Lobular inflammation including lymphocytes and plasma cells (HE × 200)

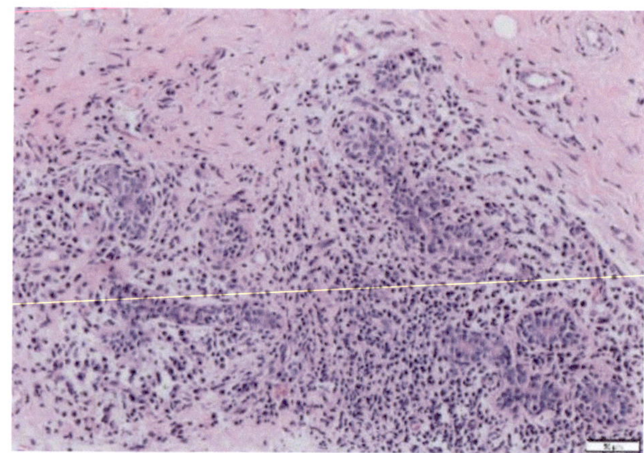

Fig. 22 Lobular inflammation including lymphocytes and plasma cells (HE × 200)

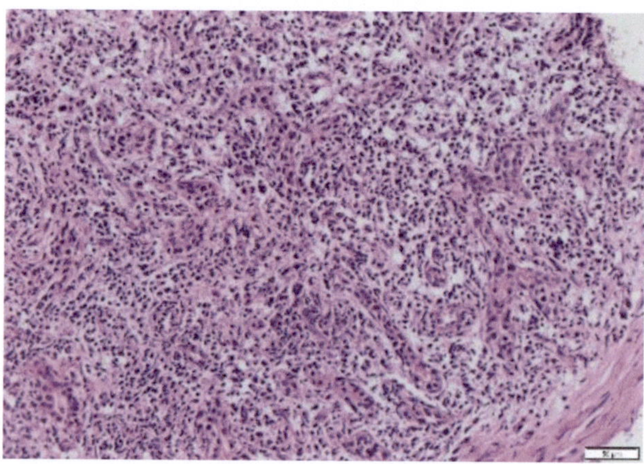

Fig. 23 Lobular inflammation including lymphocytes and plasma cells (HE × 400)

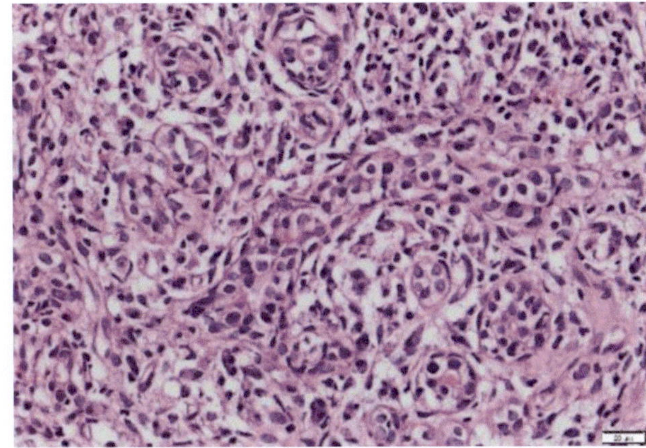

Fig. 24 Neutrophilic microabscesses (HE × 400)

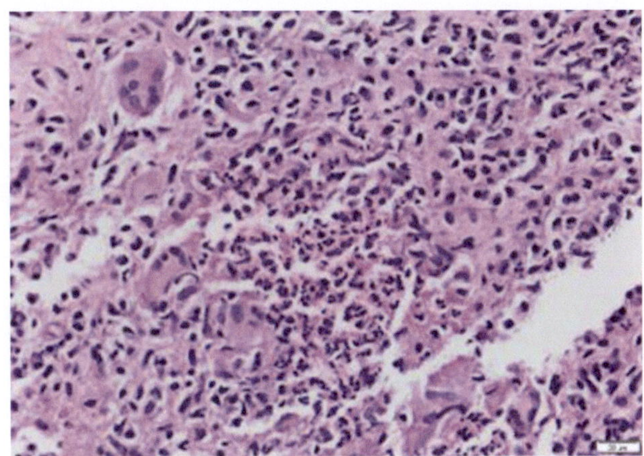

Fig. 25 A cystic space that does not contain foreign material or secretion surrounded by neutrophils (HE × 400)

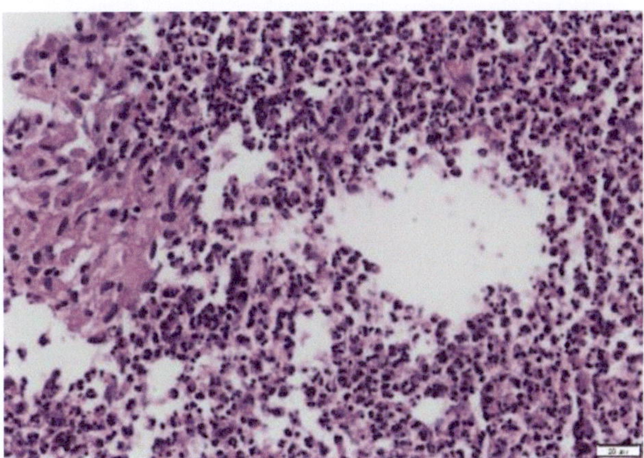

Fig. 26 Abscess formation that effaces lobules due to progressive inflammation (HE × 200)

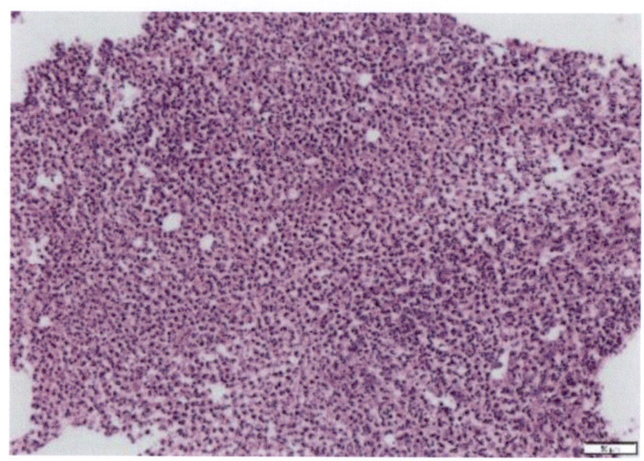

Fig. 27 Disrupted lobular architecture by AE1/AE3 stain (×200)

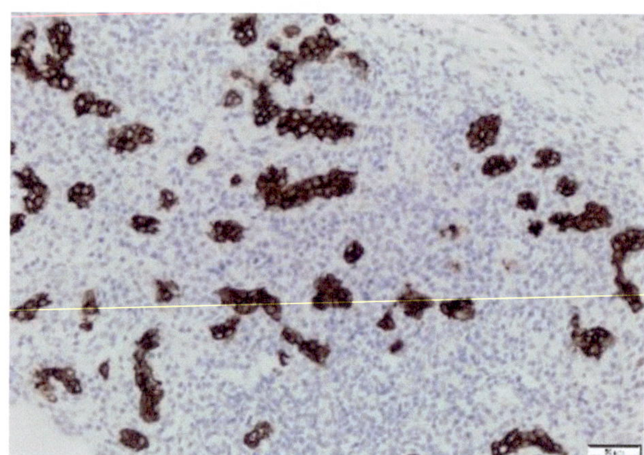

Fig. 28 CD68-positive epithelioid cells and multinucleated giant cells (×100)

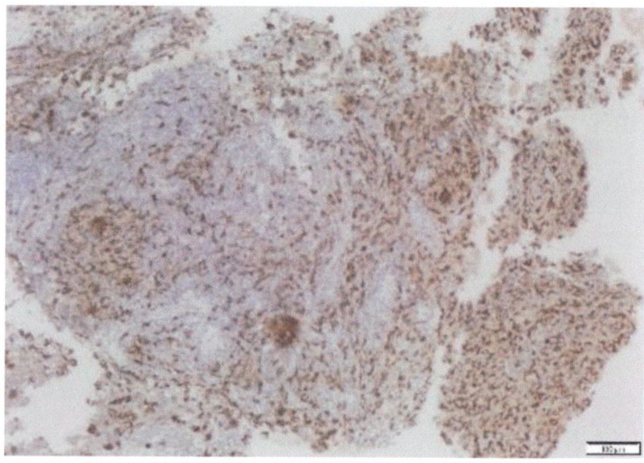

4 Ancillary Diagnostic Studies

Gram stain for bacteria, Ziehl-Neelsen for tuberculosis, PAS, and methenamine silver stain for fungal infection provide exclusion of infectious causes of granulomatous inflammation.

Determining T cell predominance, immunohistochemistry for T and B markers may be useful [16].

References

1. Milward TM, Gough MH. Granulomatous lesions in the breast presenting as carcinoma. Surg Gynecol Obstet. 1970;130:478–82.
2. Cohen C. Granulomatous mastitis. A review of 5 cases. S Afr Med J. 1977;52:14–6.
3. Kessler E, Wolloch Y. Granulomatous mastitis: a lesion clinically simulating carcinoma. Am J Clin Pathol. 1972;58:642–6. https://doi.org/10.1093/ajcp/58.6.642.
4. Nemenqani D, Yaqoob N, Hafiz M. Fine needle aspiration cytology of granulomatous mastitis with special emphasis on microbiologic correlation. Acta Cytol. 2009;53:667–71. https://doi.org/10.1159/000325408.
5. Nemenqani D, Yaqoob N. Fine needle aspiration cytology of inflammatory breast lesions. J Pak Med Assoc. 2009;59:167–70.
6. Seo HR, Na KY, Yim HE, Kim TH, Kang DK, Oh KK, et al. Differential diagnosis in idiopathic granulomatous mastitis and tuberculous mastitis. J Breast Cancer. 2012;15:111–8. https://doi.org/10.4048/jbc.2012.15.1.111.
7. Tse GM, Poon CS, Law BK, Pang LM, Chu WC, Ma TK. Fine needle aspiration cytology of granulomatous mastitis. J Clin Pathol. 2003;56:519–21. https://doi.org/10.1136/jcp.56.7.519.
8. Ail DA, Bhayekar P, Joshi A, Pandya N, Nasare A, Lengare P, et al. Clinical and cytological spectrum of granulomatous mastitis and utility of FNAC in picking up tubercular mastitis: an eight-year study. J Clin Diagn Res. 2017;11:EC45-EC49. https://doi.org/10.7860/JCDR/2017/25635.9591.
9. Chandanwale S, Naragude P, Shetty A, Sawadkar M, Raj A, Bhide A, et al. Cytomorphological spectrum of granulomatous mastitis: a study of 33 cases. Eur J Breast Health. 2020;16:146–51. https://doi.org/10.5152/ejbh.2020.5185.
10. Gangopadhyay M, De A, Chakrabarti I, Ray S, Giri A, Das R. Idiopathic granulomatous mastitis-utility of fine needle aspiration cytology (FNAC) in preventing unnecessary surgery. J Turk Ger Gynecol Assoc. 2010;11:127–30. https://doi.org/10.5152/jtgga.2010.18.
11. Helal TE, Shash LS, Saad El-Din SA, Saber SM. Idiopathic granulomatous mastitis: cytologic and histologic study of 65 Egyptian patients. Acta Cytol. 2016;60:438–44. https://doi.org/10.1159/000448800.
12. Yip CH, Jayaram G, Swain M. The value of cytology in granulomatous mastitis: a report of 16 cases from Malaysia. Aust N Z J Surg. 2000;70:103–5. https://doi.org/10.1046/j.1440-1622.2000.01764.x.
13. Kaur AC, Dal H, Müezzinoğlu B, Paksoy N. Idiopathic granulomatous mastitis. Report of a case diagnosed with fine needle aspiration cytology. Acta Cytol. 1999;43:481–4. https://doi.org/10.1159/000331104.
14. Hoda SA. Inflammatory and reactive tumors. In: Hoda SA, Koerner FC, Brogi E, Rosen PP, editors. Rosens's breast pathology. 4th ed. Philadelphia: Wolters Kluwer; 2015a. p. 37–77.
15. Hoda SA. Inflammatory and reactive tumors. In: Hoda SA, Koerner FC, Brogi E, Rosen PP, editors. Rosens's breast pathology. 4th ed. Philadelphia: Wolters Kluwer; 2015b. p. 79–94.

16. Erhan Y, Veral A, Kara E, Ozdemir N, Kapkac M, Ozdedeli E, et al. A clinicopathologic study of a rare clinical entity mimicking breast carcinoma: idiopathic granulomatous mastitis. Breast. 2000;9:52–6. https://doi.org/10.1054/brst.1999.0072.
17. Jiang L, Li X, Sun B, Ma T, Kong X, Yang Q. Clinicopathological features of granulomatous lobular mastitis and mammary duct ectasia. Oncol Lett. 2020;19:840–8. https://doi.org/10.3892/ol.2019.11156.
18. Allen SG, Soliman AS, Toy K, Omar OS, Youssef T, Karkouri M, et al. Chronic mastitis in Egypt and Morocco: differentiating between idiopathic granulomatous mastitis and IgG4-related disease. Breast J. 2016;22:501–9. https://doi.org/10.1111/tbj.12628.
19. Memis A, Bilgen I, Ustun EE, Ozdemir N, Erhan Y, Kapkac (2002) Granulomatous mastitis: imaging findings with histopathologic correlation. Clin Radiol 57: 1001–1006. https://doi.org/10.1053/crad.2002.1056.

Pathological Differential Diagnoses for Granulomatous Mastitis

Shyamala Fernandez (iD)

1 Granulomatous Mastitis

Granulomatous mastitis can be idiopathic or secondary to numerous underlying etiologies such as infective causes (tuberculosis and fungi), sarcoidosis, Wegener's granulomatosis, complication of diabetes (diabetic mastopathy), and silicone implants to name a few.

2 Idiopathic Granulomatous Mastitis

Occurs in premenopausal women (can occur 2 up to 6 years after pregnancy). It is uncommon in males and pregnancy [1].

Presenting symptom is usually a palpable mass which is sometimes tender.

Macroscopic description: ill-defined mass.

Microscopic description: lobulocentric noncaseating granulomas with/without microabscesses; no foreign body is identified. Ziehl-Neelson and PAS for acid-fast bacilli and fungi are negative.

This is a diagnosis of exclusion.

S. Fernandez (✉)
Department of Pathology, Ealing Hospital, London North West University Healthcare NHS Trust, London, UK
e-mail: shyamala.fernandez@nhs.net

3 Differential Diagnoses for Granulomatous Mastitis

3.1 Breast Infarct

Infarction of the breast is seen more commonly in the third trimester of pregnancy or 6 weeks postpartum. Tends to be seen in lactating breast. Infarcted fibroadenoma and papillomas can also occur in nonpregnant women. Extensive infarction or necrosis of the breast is uncommon and often associated with warfarin therapy.

3.1.1 Macroscopic Description

Circumscribed area of necrosis.

3.1.2 Microscopic Description

Necrosis with surrounding acute inflammation and fibroblastic proliferation (Fig. 1). Inflammation (vasculitis) as well as thrombotic blood vessels.

3.2 Xanthogranulomatous Mastitis (Fat Necrosis)

3.2.1 Macroscopic Description

Yellow discoloration of fat associated with fibrosis. There may be cyst formation and calcification.

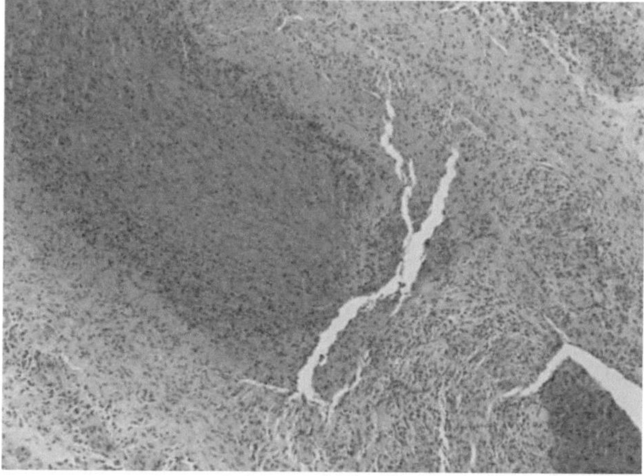

Fig. 1 Coagulation necrosis with inflamed granulation tissue (HE × 200)

3.2.2 Microscopic Description

Abundant lipid-laden as well as foamy macrophages surrounding cystic spaces, fatty cysts, and cholesterol clefts (Fig. 2).

Foreign-body-type multinucleate histiocytes, lymphocytes, and plasma cells.

Older lesions show collagen and fibroblastic proliferation (Fig. 3).

Fibrosis/scarring and calcification (late stage).

Immunohistochemistry Histiocytes show CD68 positivity and are negative for cytokeratins (AE1/AE3, MNF116, CAM 5.2) as well as S100.

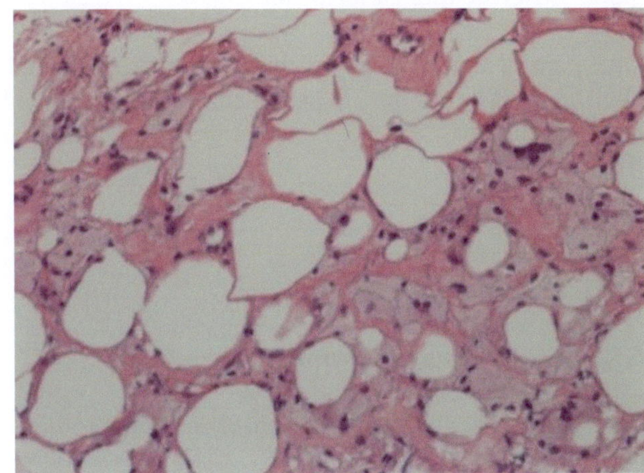

Fig. 2 Fat necrosis with foamy histiocytes and fatty cysts (HE × 400)

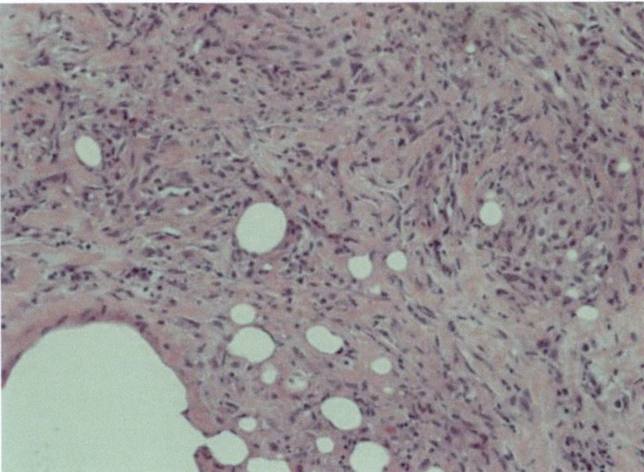

Fig. 3 Fibroblastic proliferation and collagen deposition (HE × 200)

3.3 Plasma Cell Mastitis

Can occur quite some time after the woman ceases breastfeeding. Presentation includes nipple discharge, erythema of the breast, and mastalgia.

3.3.1 Macroscopic Description

Duct ectasia containing viscous cream material.

3.3.2 Microscopic Description

Dilatation of the breast ducts with extensive lymphoplasmacytic infiltrate around ducts as well as lobules, hyperplasia of the ductal epithelium, necrosis, and scattered granulomas as well as histiocytes (xanthogranulomatous inflammation) (Fig. 4).

3.4 Periductal Mastitis

3.4.1 Macroscopic Description

Breast tissue showing white fibrous areas with prominent cystic structures containing viscous material.

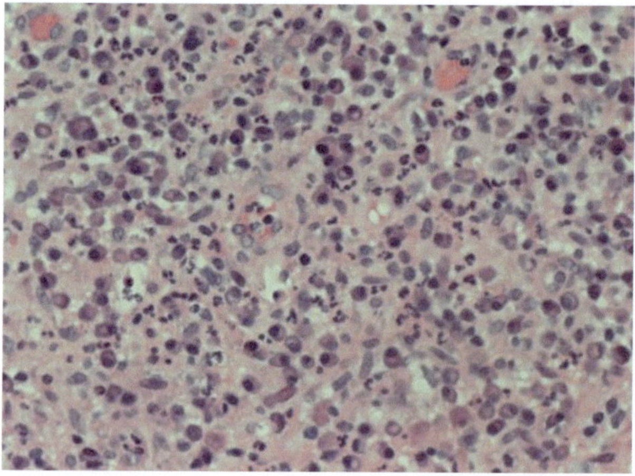

Fig. 4 Plasma cell mastitis (HE × 400)

Fig. 5 Dilated breast duct with surrounding chronic inflammation and fibrosis (HE × 200)

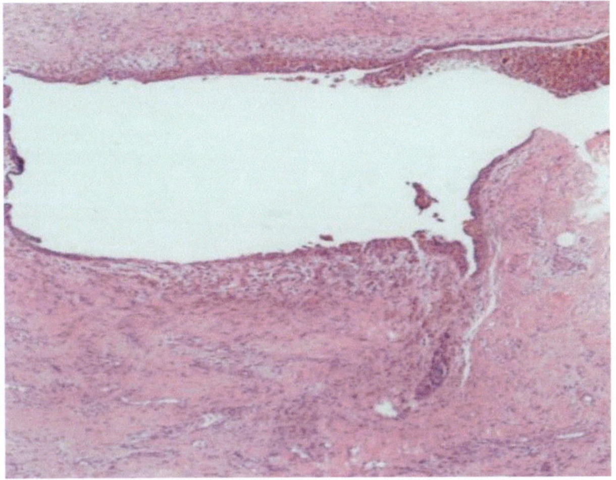

3.4.2 Microscopic Description

Duct ectasia with surrounding periductal chronic inflammation (Fig. 5).

3.5 Cystic Neutrophilic Granulomatous Mastitis

Rare subtype of mastitis caused by bacteria (*Corynebacterium* species) [2].

3.5.1 Macroscopic Description

Mass with possible skin sinus.

3.5.2 Microscopic Description

Suppurative lipogranulomas comprising central lipid vacuoles with surrounding rim of polymorphs and outer cuff of epithelioid histiocytes.

3.6 Sarcoidosis

Although rarely involves the breast, it can begin in the breast and remain localized for long periods. Breast involvement may also be part of systemic disease.

Presents as single or multiple breast masses.

Fig. 6 Discrete non-necrotizing epithelioid granulomas (HE × 200)

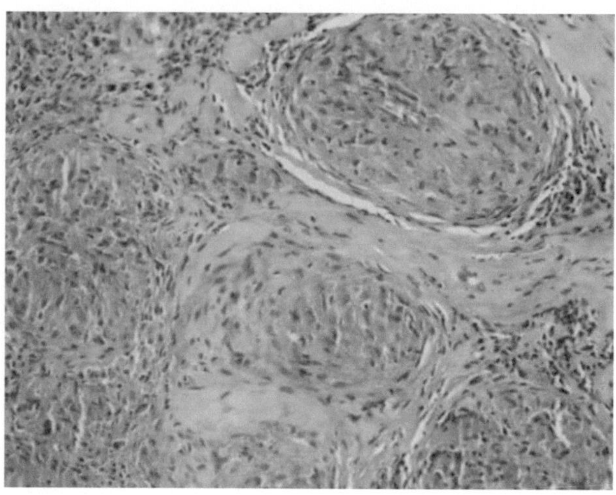

3.6.1 Macroscopic Description

Firm nodular breast tissue.

3.6.2 Microscopic Description

Discrete/"naked" non-necrotizing epithelioid granulomas with scanty lymphocytic infiltration, fibrosis, and multinucleated histiocytes which may contain asteroid bodies (star-shaped inclusions) and/or Schaumann bodies (concentrically lamellated calcified nodules). The granulomas may be lobulocentric (centered on breast lobules) or found between breast lobules. Microabscesses and central necrosis are not a feature (Fig. 6).

Many patients have history of systemic sarcoidosis (extramammary). Infective causes such as tuberculosis and fungi need to be excluded before a diagnosis of sarcoidosis can be made. Clinicopathological correlation and imaging are vital.

3.7 *Mammary Tuberculosis*

Commonly presents as mass, sinus, or a combination of the two [3].

3.7.1 Macroscopic Description

Mass with or without sinus tract.

3.7.2   Microscopic Description

Coalescing as well as non-coalescing granulomas including Langhans-type giant cells and chronic inflammatory cells are scattered throughout the breast parenchyma. Central caseating necrosis is evident along with possible bacteria within areas of necrosis. Polymorphs are present but are not a prominent feature (Figs. 7, 8, and 9).

Special stain: Ziehl-Neelson stain to identify acid-fast bacilli.

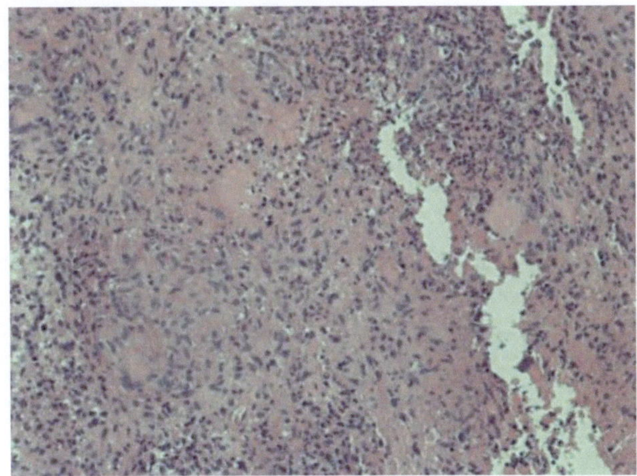

Fig. 7 Necrotizing granulomatous inflammation (HE × 200)

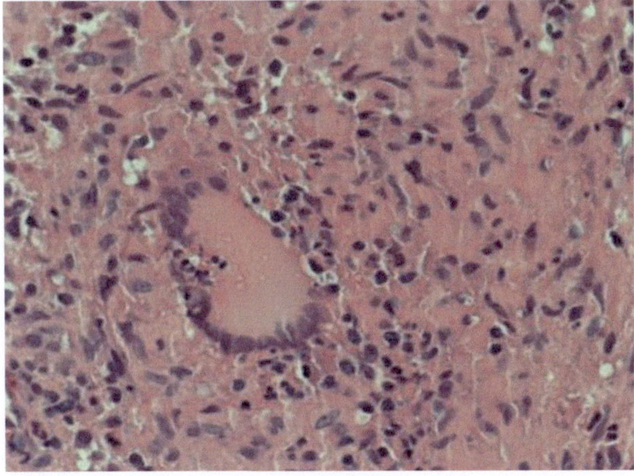

Fig. 8 Epithelioid granuloma with Langhans-type giant cell (HE × 400)

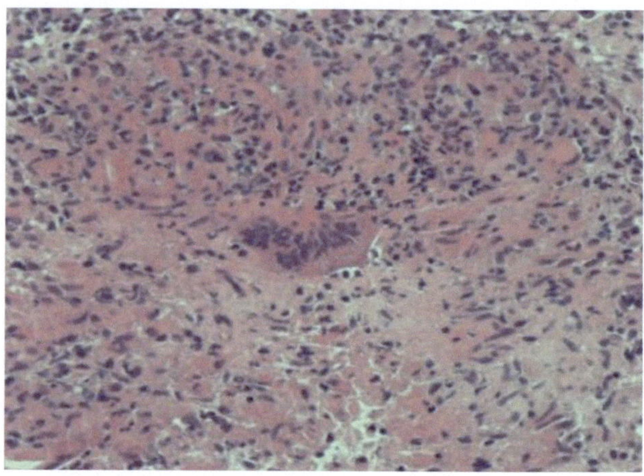

Fig. 9 Epithelioid granuloma with foreign-body-type giant cell (HE × 400)

3.8   Granulomatous Reaction in Carcinoma

Granulomatous reaction in breast carcinoma is extremely rare as it is an immune response commonly seen against infectious agents and some nonneoplastic conditions. The etiology of granulomatous reaction associated with breast cancer is unclear but may be secondary to immunologic reaction to tumor antigens.

3.8.1   Macroscopic Description

Focal asymmetric or ill-defined breast mass.

3.8.2   Microscopic Description

Granulomatous inflammation surrounding groups of breast cancer cells.

3.9   Inflammatory Pseudotumour/Inflammatory Myofibroblastic Tumor

Rare low-grade lesion of the breast. This entity remains poorly defined due to scarcity of literature.

3.9.1   Macroscopic Description

Nodular homogenous tan to yellow fibrotic tissue.

3.9.2 Microscopic Description

Mixture of myofibroblastic as well as fibroblastic cells and acute as well as chronic inflammatory cells including eosinophils. Background of abundant blood vessels.

3.10 Wegener Granulomatosis in Breast

Presenting features are tenderness and palpable (sometimes bilateral) breast lump.

3.10.1 Macroscopic Description

Sharply delineated nodules without microcalcification; necrosis is present.

3.10.2 Microscopic Description

Necrotizing granulomatous vasculitis (Fig. 10).

3.11 Lupus Mastitis

Unusual variant of systemic lupus erythematosus (SLE) or discoid lupus erythematosus (DLE).

Fig. 10 Necrotizing granulomatous inflammation with vasculitis (HE × 200)

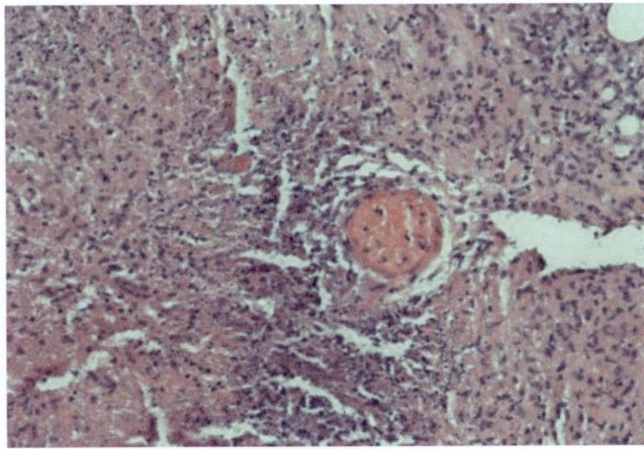

3.11.1 Macroscopic Description

Subcutaneous breast mass.

3.11.2 Microscopic Description

Inflammation of adipocytes (panniculitis) showing lobular architectures with admixed lymphoplasmacytic infiltrate including lymphoid follicles. Lymphocytic vasculitis may also be present.

Immunohistochemistry: mixed chronic inflammatory cell population comprising CD3+ as well as CD4+ T cells, CD20+ B cells, and plasma cells.

3.12 Paraffinoma (Sclerosing Lipogranuloma)

Typically caused by paraffin injection into the breast parenchyma for breast augmentation. Clinical presentation includes painless as well as painful lumps, abscess, ulceration, and discolored skin.

3.12.1 Macroscopic Description

Firm, yellow to greyish-white tissue.

3.12.2 Microscopic Description

Foreign-body-type granulomas including cholesterol clefts, foamy macrophages, and droplets of fat in breast parenchyma with minimal chronic inflammation. (Fig. 11).

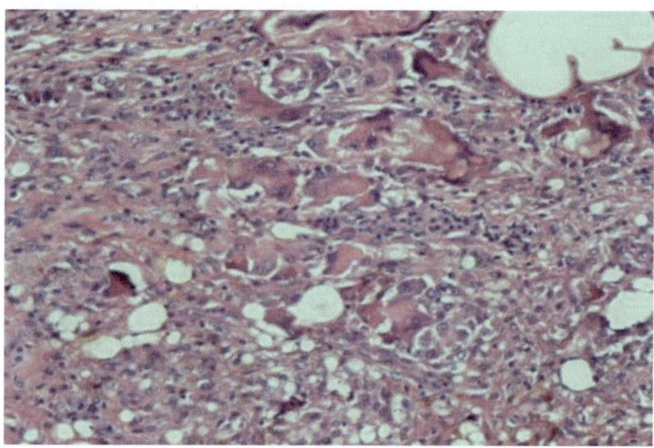

Fig. 11 Foreign body giant cell reaction (HE × 200)

3.13 Silicone Granuloma

Fibrous capsule develops around the breast implant containing silicone. Granulomatous inflammation is secondary to ruptured (extracellular) capsule [4].

3.13.1 Macroscopic Description

Nodular hard breast tissue containing cystic spaces filled with material with/without sinus tract.

3.13.2 Microscopic Description

Foreign-body-type reaction including multinucleate foreign-body-type giant cells, fibrosis, silicone within variable-size spaces like clear spaces with refractile material, and synovial hyperplasia on the surface of the implant (Figs. 12 and 13).

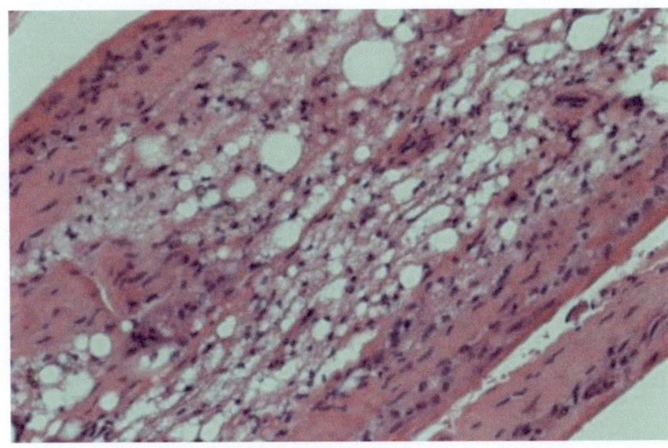

Fig. 12 Silicone granuloma in ruptured breast implant capsule (HE × 200)

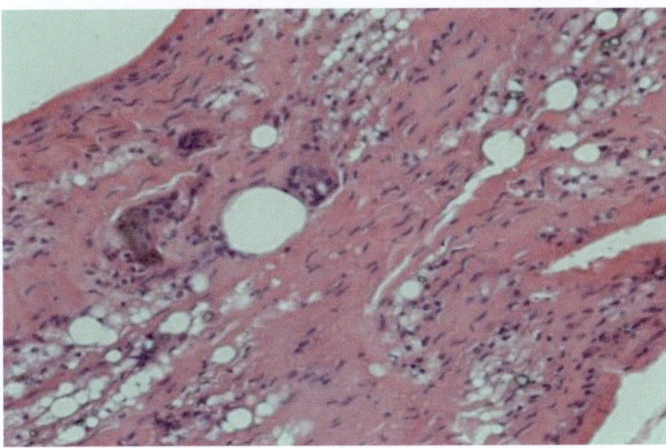

Fig. 13 Silicone granuloma with foreign-body-type giant cells (HE × 200)

3.14   Eosinophilic Mastitis

Can be associated with asthma.

3.14.1   Macroscopic Description

Breast mass.

3.14.2   Microscopic Description

Dense periductal and lobular active chronic inflammation including numerous eosinophils (Figs. 14 and 15).

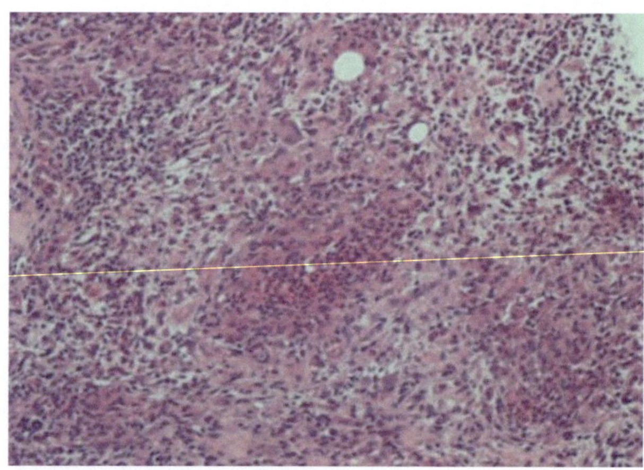

Fig. 14 Granulomatous inflammation with numerous eosinophils (HE × 200)

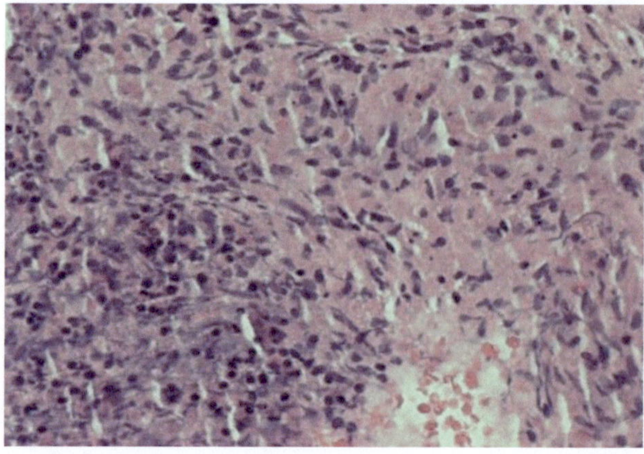

Fig. 15 Epithelioid granuloma containing numerous eosinophils (HE × 400)

3.15   Diabetic Mastopathy

Associated with type I diabetes mellitus; bilateral involvement up to 50% of cases.

3.15.1   Macroscopic Description

Irregular firm white to gray appearance.

3.15.2   Microscopic Description

Combination of compact collagenous/keloidal-like fibrosis, chronic inflammatory infiltrate, and interspersed myofibroblastic cells. Stromal mitoses are not seen (Figs. 16, 17, and 18).

Immunohistochemistry: CD20-positive lymphocytes (B-lineage).

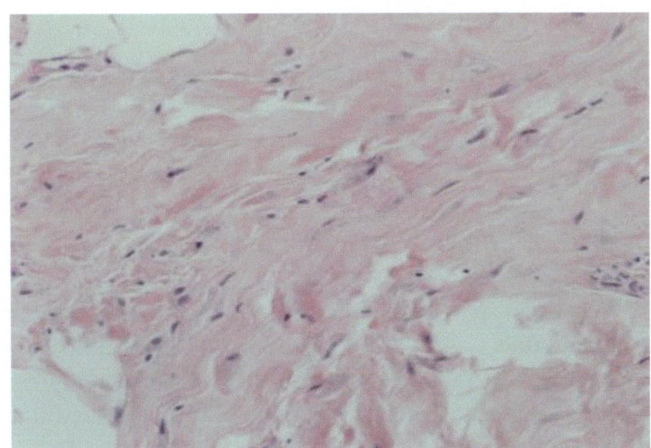

Fig. 16 Dense collagenous/keloidal fibrosis (HE × 200)

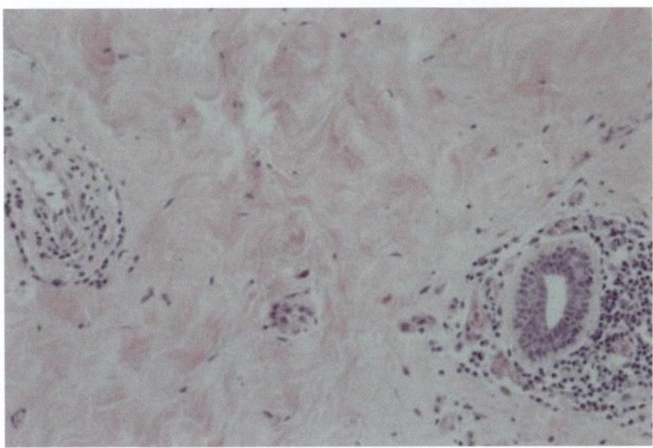

Fig. 17 Periductal and perivascular lymphocytic infiltrates (HE × 200)

Fig. 18 Stromal
myofibroblasts (HE × 400)

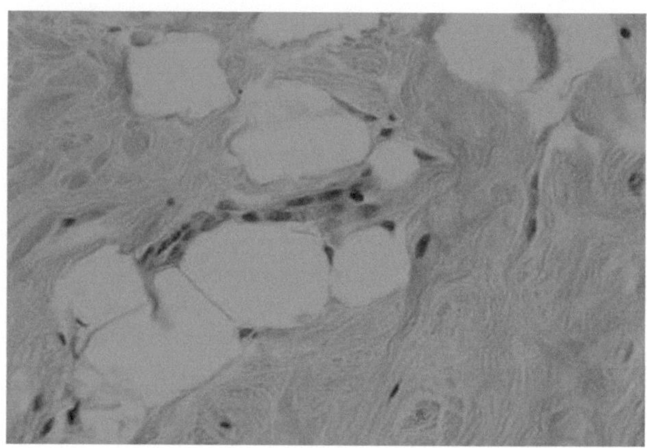

3.16   Mammary Amyloidosis

Nontender single or multiple breast lumps.

3.16.1   Macroscopic Description

Nodular pearlescent to multicolored mass.

3.16.2   Microscopic Description

Extracellular deposit staining a pink/light red color is seen in breast parenchyma. Atrophic ducts, amyloid deposit around individual adipocytes and in vessel walls, multinucleate giant cell reaction, and osseous metaplasia may also be present.

Special stain: Congo Red stain. Under polarized light, the red stain shows apple green birefringence.

3.17   IgG4-Related Sclerosing Mastitis

Uncommon benign fibroinflammatory breast lump.

3.17.1   Macroscopic Description

Mass-forming lesion.

3.17.2 Microscopic Description

Storiform fibrosis, obliterative vasculitis, and lymphoplasmacytic infiltrate rich in IgG4-positive plasma cells.

Immunohistochemistry: IgG4, CD138 (plasma cells).

3.18 Histoplasmosis

Uncommon in breast. Presents usually with multiple nonhealing ulcers.

3.18.1 Macroscopic Description

Mass with/without sinus tract.

3.18.2 Microscopic Description

Non-necrotizing histiocytic granulomatous inflammation with sinus tracts. Histoplasma spores may or may not be identified within histiocytes or in extracellular spaces (Fig. 19).

Special stains: PAS and GMS (highlight histoplasma cell wall).

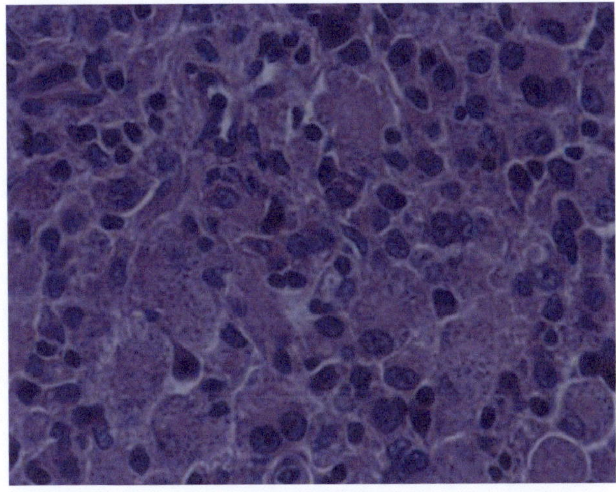

Fig. 19 Histoplasma spores within histiocytes (HE × 400)

3.19 Blastomycosis

Rare to have localized infection solely confined to the breast. Usually presents with multiple organ involvement. Can present initially as a nodular lesion with tendency to ulcerate later.

3.19.1 Macroscopic Description

Subcutaneous nodular skin lesion which may be ulcerated.

3.19.2 Microscopic Description

Granulomatous inflammation and neutrophilic infiltrates. Fungal spores within giant cells.

Special stains: PAS and GMS (identify yeasts with broad-based budding).

3.20 Cryptococcosis

Firm, nontender breast mass.

3.20.1 Macroscopic Description

Well-circumscribed, encapsulated, multilocular mass composed of gelatinous material.

3.20.2 Microscopic Description

Granulomatous inflammation with or without central necrosis and sheets of foamy macrophages can be seen. Yeast forms surrounded by edema and inflammatory reaction. Diffuse histiocytic granulomatous inflammation may be seen in patients who are immunodeficient.

Special stains: PAS, GMS, and mucicarmine (identify variably encapsulated yeasts with narrow budding).

3.21   Aspergillosis

3.21.1   Macroscopic Description

Mass with hemorrhage and abscess.

3.21.2   Microscopic Description

Necrotizing granulomatous inflammation with dichotomous branching hyphae with frequent septation.
   Special stains: PAS and GMS.

3.22   Coccidiodomycosis

3.22.1   Macroscopic Description

Mass with sinus tract.

3.22.2   Microscopic Description

Pseudoepitheliomatous hyperplasia of overlying skin and acute suppurative inflammation with variable infiltrate of polymorphs, eosinophils, histiocytes, multinucleate giant cells, plasma cells, and rarely lymphocytes. Non-necrotizing granulomatous inflammation with sinus tracts can also be a feature. Rarely, spherules in association with histiocytic neutrophilic infiltrate or within hyperplastic squamous epithelium may be seen.
   Special stains: PAS and GMS (identify large yeast forms with broad-based budding).

3.23   Filariasis

Mammary filariasis is caused by *Wuchereria bancrofti* and presents as a solitary nontender/painless unilateral breast mass, although multiple lesions can occur in a minority of cases. The lesion(s) is usually found in the subcutaneous tissue and may be fixed to the skin.

3.23.1 Macroscopic Description

Hard mass with cutaneous attachment.

3.23.2 Microscopic Description

Cross section(s) of adult filarial worm which may be well preserved or degenerate/calcified with surrounding chronic eosinophils as well as granulomatous inflammation and fibrosis.

References

1. Wikipedia (n.d.). https://en.wikipedia.org/wiki/Granulomatous_mastitis.
2. Wu JM, Turashvili G. Breast infectious cystic neutrophilic granulomatous mastitis. PathologyOutlines.com, Inc; 2020. https://www.pathologyoutlines.com/topic/breastcystic-granulomatousmastitis.html
3. Warzecha H. Breast infectious tuberculosis. PathologyOutlines.com, Inc; 2010. https://www.pathologyoutlines.com/topic/breastTB.html
4. Warzecha H. Breast inflammatory silicone leak/lymphadenopathy. PathologyOutlines.com, Inc; 2021. https://www.pathologyoutlines.com/topic/breastsiliconebreastimplants.html

Medical Treatment and Prognosis

Hande Koksal (iD)

Since idiopathic granulomatous mastitis was first described, an ideal treatment approach has not yet been established. One of the most important reasons for this is that the etiopathogenesis is not yet clearly understood and the heterogeneous clinical appearance within the patient population [1–4]. In recent years, the etiopathogenesis is based mostly on autoimmune and immune dysregulation which raises the question of whether IGM is a surgical or a systemic disease [5–9]. Consequently, the use of immunosuppressive drugs such as corticosteroids and methotrexate has increased for the treatment of IGM [10–16].

In this chapter, the treatment and management approaches of IGM and the optimal treatment options recommended are discussed in the light of the literature.

1 Treatment Approaches

Today, it is possible to examine the treatment approaches used in IGM under three main headings. These are conservative treatment approaches, surgical interventions, and combined treatment approaches (Table 1) [3, 4, 17, 18].

An optimal treatment option for IGM has not yet been established. Idiopathic granulomatous mastitis is a benign disease with chronic granulomatous inflammation. It has a very heterogeneous clinical spectrum, and therefore, it may not be correct to apply the same treatment approach to every patient. It will be much more appropriate to choose the treatment option according to the patient. Therefore, a classification for IGM is needed to determine the optimal

H. Koksal (✉)
Department of General Surgery, Selcuk University, Faculty of Medicine, Konya, Türkiye

© The Author(s), under exclusive license to Springer Nature Switzerland AG 2023
H. Koksal, N. Kadoglou (eds.), *Idiopathic Granulomatous Mastitis*,
https://doi.org/10.1007/978-3-031-30391-3_11

Table 1 Treatment approaches used until today

Treatment approaches
Conservative approaches
Wait and watch
Only antibiotics
Nonsteroidal anti-inflammatory drugs
Immunosuppressive therapy
Corticosteroid
Systemic corticosteroids
Local corticosteroid administration
Topical
Intralesional
Combine local (topical + intralesional)
Combine administration (local + systemic)
Methotrexate
Azathioprine
Mycophenolate mofetil
Traditional medicine
Others
Colchicine
Etanercept
Minocycline
Bromocriptine
Platelet-rich plasma
Surgical procedures
Drainage
Excision
Mastectomy
Combine treatment approaches
Drainage + antibiotic
Drainage + corticosteroid (systemic or local)
Excision + antibiotic
Excision + corticosteroid (systemic or local)
Drainage + excision + antibiotic
Drainage + excision + corticosteroid (systemic or local)

personalized treatment approach. Two clinical classifications have been proposed for IGM [19–21] and these classifications proposed by Irkorucu [20] and Yaghan et al. [21] are similar. While the classification proposed by Irkorucu [20] can be used for all granulomatous mastitis, the classification suggested by Yaghan et al. [21] is a clinically based classification of IGM. Recently, Kaviani and Vasigh [22] proposed a classification system which has the subtitle of extramammarian manifestations (see Chap. 5).

1.1 Conservative Approaches

1.1.1 Wait and Watch

Idiopathic granulomatous mastitis is a chronic granulomatous inflammation around the lobules that can be self-limiting and resolving [4, 17, 23–25].

Lai et al. [25] reported that four of eight patients with IGM who did not undergo any surgical intervention had spontaneous remission on an average of 14.5 months (range, 2 to 24 months) and no recurrence was observed on long-term follow-up.

Bouton et al. [23] analyzed 37 IGM patients retrospectively, 36 of whom were Hispanic. Thirty-two (86%) of these patients were uninsured. In this study, 27 patients were followed up without excision and the disease was found to be resolved. However, drainage and/or antibiotic treatment was applied to patients who did not undergo excision. The resolution times of lesions were found to be 0–6 months in 11 patients (41%), 6–12 months in 12 patients (44%), and > 12 months in four patients (15%). The mean time for resolution of these patients was 7.4 months (range, 0–20 months). Recurrence was observed in only three patients (8%). The authors found that the lesions could resolve spontaneously with observation. In addition, they emphasized that their findings suggest that management of IGM with close observation is feasible in some selected patients.

In the study by Davis et al. [24], 120 patients with IGM were analyzed retrospectively. Most of the patients (92%) were Hispanic. Antibiotics were prescribed to 35 patients (29%) and analgesics to 27 patients (23%). While no incision or drainage was required in 87 patients (72%), one incision or drainage was performed in 21 patients and more than one incision or drainage in 12 patients (10%). The authors reported that the lesions resolved with observation in 112 patients and the resolution times ranged between 0 and 20 months (mean: 5.1 months). About two-thirds of patients recovered in the first 6 months, 23% between 6 and 12 months, and 5% in more than 12 months. The relapse rate in this study was 16%.

In the study by Cetinkaya et al. [26], 118 IGM patients were analyzed retrospectively. Their treatment schemes were no treatment ($n = 50$, 42.4%), corticosteroid treatment ($n = 36$, 30.5%), antibiotics ($n = 21$, 17.8%), excision ($n = 9$, 7.6%), and azathioprine ($n = 2$, 1.4%). Varying numbers of drainage were applied to 54 patients. While the recovery time of patients without any treatment ranged between 1.3 and 13.8 months (mean recovery time: 5.1 months), this period varied between 0.8 and 9.8 months (mean recovery time: 3.9 months) in patients receiving corticosteroid treatment. Interestingly, there was no statistically significant difference between patients without any treatment and those who received corticosteroid treatment by means of recovery times. The authors found recurrence in 14 patients (11.9%) in their study. Considering the initial treatment of patients with recurrence, 8 patients (57.1%) had corticosteroid treatment, 4 patients (28.5%) had antibiotics, 1 patient (7.1%) was given no treatment, and 1 patient (7.1%) underwent excision. In conclusion, this study emphasized that in case of an abscess or collection, it is appropriate to give a chance to the self-limiting nature of the disease with the addition of drainage and antibiotic therapy.

In our previous study [17], it was observed that 11 of 134 IGM patients did not receive any treatment and only one patient relapsed (9%). This suggests that although the number of patients included in this group is small, a wait-and-watch approach may be an option in selected IGM patients.

In conclusion, it should be kept in mind that IGM can be self-limited and can resolve spontaneously. However, if a wait-and-watch approach is to be applied, the patient should be well informed and possible increased recovery time should be explained. The wait-and-watch strategy may be a good alternative approach for patients whose lesion size does not exceed 2 cm in patterns A and B according to the classification suggested by Yaghan et al. [21].

1.1.2 Antibiotics Only

The role of antibiotics for the treatment of IGM could not be clearly established yet [4, 27]. It is important that the clinical presentations of IGM are very heterogeneous. The general approach to the treatment of IGM is the use of antibiotics, especially in patients with signs of inflammation or an abscess-like appearance [3].

Failure to recognize the microbiological cause is an important problem in patients who have signs of inflammation on the skin or have an abscess-like appearance [17]. Kıvılcım et al. [28] investigated the bacteria mentioned in the study using a universal DNA primer in paraffin blocks of patients with IGM. The authors concluded that bacteriological agents are not the primary cause of IGM etiology.

The most comprehensive study on the use of antibiotics for IGM treatment is the study of Aghajanzadeh et al. [29]. They used antibiotics such as cloxacillin, cephalexin, ciprofloxacin, or clindamycin to treat all of their patients for approximately 3 weeks, but in only 3% of the patients, an improvement in symptoms and signs was seen.

A study by Li [30] reviewed 75 IGM patients. Thirty-one of these patients had a history of antibiotic use before admission. While 23 of these patients who received antibiotic treatment did not respond to antibiotics, eight patients were observed to have a partial response. Pathogenic microorganisms could complicate IGM and the study emphasized that the use of antibiotics may partially improve at least these symptoms or signs.

The ideal approach to the use of antibiotics is to document the potential microorganism. However, since this is not possible in IGM, empirical antibiotics are generally used. The most preferred antibiotics are cloxacillin, cephalexin, clindamycin, flucloxacillin, ciprofloxacin, or doxycycline, which are effective for gram-positive cocci [3, 29]. Apart from that, the use of rifampicin and azithromycin has also been reported in the literature [31–33].

In conclusion, although the microorganism cannot be documented in patients with IGM, considering that IGM may be complicated secondarily by a pathogenic microorganism emphasized by Li [30], empirical antibiotic treatment can be used especially in patients with signs of inflammation in the skin or with abscess-like lesions.

1.1.3   Nonsteroidal Anti-Inflammatory Drugs

In IGM, the use of corticosteroids has increased in recent years and it brings to mind the use of nonsteroidal anti-inflammatory drugs (NSAIDs) for the treatment of IGM. However, experience with the use of NSAIDs in patients with IGM is very little compared with corticosteroids [34–38].

Studies with NSAIDs as a treatment of IGM by Kaviani et al. [36, 37] are very instructive. Kaviani et al. [36] evaluated 20 IGM patients between 2007 and 2011. All patients used empirical antibiotics (at least 2 weeks) and NSAIDs (at least 2 months). They used corticosteroids for resistant or early relapse patients. They achieved excellent or good control in 15 out of 20 patients. Two patients needed corticosteroids. In another study by Kaviani et al. [37], NSAIDs were preferred as the first line for the treatment of 41.8% of 374 IGM patients. The most used NSAID in this study was naproxen. In the treatment of patients with NSAIDs, 31.5% had a *complete response* and 59.2% a *moderate response*, while 6.2% of patients did not respond to treatment, and 3.1% of patients progressed. The recurrence rate was 16.9%. The authors achieved dramatic and acceptable response to NSAIDs, although NSAIDs have been used in moderate and severe IGM patients. They emphasized that NSAIDS were as effective as prednisolone in moderate to severe cases.

In conclusion, when deciding the treatment option for a patient with IGM, if there are contradictions to the possible side effects of corticosteroids and other immunosuppressive drugs, any NSAID treatment may be used once approved by a rheumatologist. In addition, the use of NSAIDs in IGM treatment is a good research topic requiring further studies.

1.1.4   Immunosuppressive Treatment

Corticosteroids

Recently, DeHertogh et al. [39] first described the increasing interest in corticosteroid therapy for the treatment of IGM.

According to the application methods of corticosteroids in IGM treatment, it can be classified under three main headings: systemic, local (topical, intralesional, or both), or combined (systemic and local) corticosteroid therapy.

Systemic Corticosteroid Therapy

Nowadays, since DeHertogh et al. [39] first used systemic corticosteroids for the treatment of IGM, there has been an increasing interest on the use of corticosteroids for IGM treatment ([11, 15, 25, 32, 34, 37, 38, 40–75]).

Firstly, DeHertogh et al. [39] administered prednisone at a dose of 60 mg/day in an IGM patient. At the end of 3 weeks, the lesions resolved, and the treatment lasted approximately 4 months. They reported no recurrence in the patient but did not provide any information with regards to the possible side effects of corticosteroid in their article.

To date, corticosteroid therapy in IGM treatment has mostly been related to systemic corticosteroid therapy by oral application. Some of these studies or case report(s) are summarized in Table 2. As shown in this table, most corticosteroids used were intermediate acting such as prednisone, prednisolone, or methylprednisolone. Dexamethasone, a long-acting corticosteroid, was used in only two publications [43, 73]. In both publications, dexamethasone was preferred as a loading drug and the treatment was continued with prednisolone. If dexamethasone in these two studies was ignored, prednisone or prednisolone was the most used drugs.

Table 2 Summary of some studies using only systemic corticosteroid therapy in IGM treatment

Author(s)	Drug and dose	Duration of treatment	Recovery time	Recurrence	Side effect(s)
Atak et al. [42]	Methylprednisolone – 0.8 mg/kg/days – Tapered down each week at a rate of 0.1 mg/kg/day	8 wks	Unkn	No	Unkn
Binesh et al. [43] The patient with arthritis and erythema nodosum	– Dexamethasone 12 mg/day (1.5 days) – After that, prednisolone 30 mg/day – After 1 week the dose was halved and slowly tapered	Unkn	Unkn	No	Unkn
Boufettal et al. [34]	Prednisone 1 mg/kg per day for 2 months with gradual dose reduction	2 mos	Unkn	4/5 patients	Unkn
Casteren et al. [44]	Patient 1, methylprednisolone – 32 mg/day (2 wks) – 16 mg/day, (2 wks) – 8 mg/day, (2 wks)	6 wks	2 wks	No	Hot flushes Some nausea
Cetin et al. [10]	Methylprednisolone – 0.8 mg/kg/day – tapered slowly according to the clinical and radiological response		11.7 ± 5.5 wks (4–24 wks)	20.7%	Weight gain Hirsutism Iatrogenic Cushing
Chirappapha et al. [46]	Corticosteroid (dose unknown)	Unkn	114.5 days (42–416)	1/6 patients	Unkn
DeHertogh et al. [39]	Patient: prednisone 60 mg/day	4 mos	3 wks	No	Unkn

(continued)

Table 2 (continued)

Author(s)	Drug and dose	Duration of treatment	Recovery time	Recurrence	Side effect(s)
Deng et al. [47]	Prednisolone – 30 mg/day, (the 1st and 2nd wks) – 20 mg/day, (the 3rd wk) – 10 mg/day, (the 4th wk) – 5 mg/day, the 5th and 6th wks	Unkn	1.5 Mos (1.5–9)	18.5%	Unkn
Erozgen et al. [48]	Prednisolone – 32 mg/day, (2 wks) – Tapered in 2 mos	2.5 mos	Unkn	1/25 patients (4%)	Weight gain
Gopalakrishnan Nair et al. [49]	Prednisolone – Loading dose of 0.5 mg/kg – Tapered to maintenance dose of 5 mg/day, by 4 weeks – Maintenance dose for 6 mos	7 mos	Unkn	1/23 patients (4.3%)	Unkn
Goulabchand et al. [50]	Patient: Prednisone – 35 mg/day (1 mo) – Tapered in 3 mos	4 mos	Nearly 1 mo	No	Unkn
Hashmi et al. [52]	Patient: Prednisolone – 20 mg/day	Unkn	Unkn	Unsuccessful	Unkn
Hwang et al. [54]	Patient: Prednisolone – 40 mg/day	2 wks	2 wks	Unsuccessful	Unkn
Karanlik et al. [55]	Methylprednisolone – 0.5 mg/day (2–4 wks) – Then tapered down slowly for 4 wks	Unkn	Unkn	30%	Cushingoid appearance Hirsutism

(continued)

Table 2 (continued)

Author(s)	Drug and dose	Duration of treatment	Recovery time	Recurrence	Side effect(s)
Katz et al. [56]	Patient 1: Prednisone 40 mg/day (Treatment was changed to methotrexate) Patient 2: Prednisone 40 mg/day Patient 3: Prednisone 30 mg/day Patient 4: Prednisone 20 mg/day	10 days Unkn 1 year Unkn	6 wks Unkn Unkn	No No Yes (dose at 5 mg/days	Corticosteroid-induced diabetes mellitus No No No
Kaviani et al. [37]	Prednisolone (dose unknown)	Unkn	13.9 ± 10.4 wks	24.8%	Unkn
Mahmodlou et al. [59]	Prednisolone – 100 mg/day (2 wks) – 50 mg/day (2 wks) – 25 mg/day (2 wks) – 10 mg/day (2 wks) – 5 mg/day (1 wk)	9 wks	Unkn	3/33 patients (nearly 9%)	Weight gain Acne
Montazer et al. [15]	Prednisolone – Low dose (5 mg/day) – High dose – 50 mg/day (3 days) – 25 mg/day (3 days) – 12.5 mg/day (3 days) – 5 mg/days (afterwards)	2 months	3.25 ± 1.75 mos 5.28 ± 3.93 mos	37.5% 0%	Unkn
Mizrakli et al. [38]	Prednisolone (dose unknown)	Unkn	Unkn	No	Unkn
Naraynsingh et al. [62]	Prednisolone – Patient 1: 60 mg/day – Patient 2: 80 mg/day	Unkn Unkn	8 wks 6 wks	No No	Unkn Unkn

(continued)

Table 2 (continued)

Author(s)	Drug and dose	Duration of treatment	Recovery time	Recurrence	Side effect(s)
Néel et al. [63]	Corticosteroid 40 mg/day, (20–60 mg/day)	15 mos (4–117)	Unkn	46%	Unkn
Olsen and Dilaveri [64]	Corticosteroid (dose unknown)	Unkn	Unkn	Unsuccessful	Unkn
Oran et al. [65]	Prednisolone – 32 mg/day, (2 wks) – Tapered in 6 wks	Nearly 2 mos	Unkn	5/25 patients (20%)	No
Pandey et al. [66]	Prednisone – 40 mg/day (2–4 wks) – tapered by 5–10 mg every 2–4 weeks based on symptom relief	Unkn	159 days Q1 = 120 days Q3 = 241 days	23%	Unkn
Ruiter et al. [67]	Patient: Prednisone – 60 mg/day (2 wks) – Tapered to 20 mg/day (6 wks) – 2.5 mg/wk. – Tapered in 5 mos	5 mos	2 Mos	Yes	Moon face Weight gain
Sakurai et al. [68]	Prednisolone 60 mg/day	7.5 mos (1–10)	4–10 Mos	1/8 patients	
Salehi et al. [32]	Prednisolone – 60 mg/day (2 wks) – 40 mg/day (8 wks) – Tapered for 6 mos	8 Mos	Unkn	6.2%	
Sheybani et al. [70]	Prednisone – 0.5–1 mg/kg/day (3–4 weeks) – 5.0 mg per week until prednisone tapered to 10.0–15.0 mg/day – Continue with more slow taper by 5.0 mg every 2–3 weeks until treatment is discontinued	Unkn	Unkn	20% (tapering period)	
Skandarajah et al. [71]	Prednisolone 0.5 mg/kg/day	Unkn	3 mos (2–24)	4/8 patients	

(continued)

Table 2 (continued)

Author(s)	Drug and dose	Duration of treatment	Recovery time	Recurrence	Side effect(s)
Su et al. [72]	Patient 1, prednisolone – 0.6 mg/kg/day (28 days) – Tapered in 3 wks	1.5 Mos	1 mo	Yes	
Wang et al. [73]	Dexamethasone 5 mg/day (5 days) Prednisolone – 20 mg/day (1 wk) – 15 mg/day (1 wk) – 10 mg/day (1 wk) – So on, until treatment cessation	Unkn	258 days	22.7%	
Yabanoglu et al. [74]	Methylprednisolone – 0.8 mg/kg/day (1 Wk) – Thereafter 0.1 mg/kg/day	Unkn	6 Mos (1–15 Mos)	9/44 patients (nearly 20%)	
Yilmaz et al. [75]	Methylprednisolone – 30 mg/days (3 mos) – Tapered in 3 days	3 Mos	Unkn	12.6%	
Yuksekdag [76]	Prednisolone – 64 mg/day (4 wks) – Tapered in 2 wks	6 wks	6 wks (1–10)	14.9%	No

mo(s), month(s); wk(s), week(s); unkn, unknown; w, with; w/o, without

Low or high doses of corticosteroid was preferred depending on the type of corticosteroid. Preferred doses for prednisolone range from 20 to 80 mg/day, but the initiating dose is often around 0.5–1 mg/kg/day. The dosage of prednisone was also similar. The initiating dose for methylprednisolone was 0.5–0.8 mg/kg/day. After the initial dose, tapering and discontinuation was applied according to the clinical and/or radiological response.

There are some questions that need to be answered in systemic corticosteroid therapy.

(i) "Should systemic corticosteroids be used in every IGM patient?" The answer to this question is probably "No," given that a watch-and-wait strategy is a good approach in some IGM patients [26].

(ii) "Considering patients who recur during corticosteroid dose tapering or very soon after cessation, is there a need for maintenance corticosteroid therapy? If so, how long should this period be?" Systemic corticosteroids may be a treatment option in patterns C and D in the classification of Yaghan et al. [21], or types II, III, and IV in the classification of Irkorucu [19, 20]. If recurrences occur during cessation or after the termination of therapy, the drug doses can be reduced by spreading it over a longer period of time or combined corticosteroid therapy regimens can be used.

(iii) "What about the side effects associated with corticosteroids?" The side effects of corticosteroids are well documented. Reported side effects were weight gain, hot flashes, nausea, hirsutism, Cushing syndrome, moon face, acne, hyperglycemia or diabetes mellitus, and poor sleep [10, 44, 48, 55, 56, 59, 67, 70, 73].

In conclusion, systemic corticosteroid therapy is a good treatment option in some selected patients with IGM. Given as a single dose, early in the morning, it does not suppress the circadian peak in cortisol secretion in the next morning. In order to minimize systemic steroid-related side effects, corticosteroid treatment should be given as a single dose between 06.00 and 07.00 in the morning after breakfast.

Local Corticosteroid Therapy

Topical Corticosteroid Therapy

Altintoprak [77] successfully applied topical corticosteroid treatment in IGM. The author noted that low-dose prednisolone (30 mg/day) and topical Prednasinolone pomade (twice a day, four times per week) were administered because of the patient's peptic ulcer history. The author reported that the patient was in remission in the fifth week of the treatment, but recurrence occurred after 8 weeks. It was stated that topical corticosteroid treatment application to this patient was successful and no other recurrence was observed again.

In another study of the same center [78], they applied topical corticosteroids (twice a day, on alternate days for 4 days, with a subsequent interval of 3 days, for 12 weeks) to 11 IGM patients. All patients were successfully treated, recurrence developed in only two patients at the fifth and eighth months. These patients were also treated with topical corticosteroids. In another retrospective study from the same center, the effectiveness of topical corticosteroid treatment was again proven successful [79].

Cetin et al. [10] conducted a very important randomized, prospective study on topical corticosteroid therapy for the treatment of IGM. Moreover, 124 IGM patients were evaluated and divided into three groups according to treatment approaches: systemic corticosteroid treatment (0.8 mg/kg/day per oral), topical corticosteroid treatment (Prednasinolone 0.125% pomade, twice a day in weekdays), and combined corticosteroid treatment (0.4 mg/kg/day per oral + Prednasinolone 0.125% pomade, twice a day in weekdays). They found that the outcomes of all treatment groups were similar and the lowest corticosteroid-related side effects were observed in the topical corticosteroid group. In addition, they concluded, "topical steroids would be among first-line treatment options of IGM."

Intralesional Corticosteroid Therapy

Recently, a new application of local corticosteroids, intralesional corticosteroids, has been described for the treatment of IGM [80–82].

Alper et al. [80] administered methylprednisolone acetate, a depo-corticosteroid, and injected into the perilesional fibroglandular tissue. They achieved a complete response in 89.3% of their patients and a partial response in 10.7%, with no steroid-related side effects.

Kornfeld and Mitchell [81] administered 40 mg/1 mL triamcinolone, an intermediate-acting drug, mixed with 3 mL 2% lidocaine into the affected areas of the breast in a 7-month pregnant woman. The authors concluded that intralesional injection of steroid can provide significant symptomatic relief to patients.

In Toktas et al.'s [82] study comparing a systemic corticosteroid group with an intralesional steroid injection with concomitant topical steroid group, the complete or partial response rates of groups were 71.9% and 93.5%, respectively. The recurrence rates of the groups were 46.9% and 8.7%, respectively. Also, the corticosteroid-related side effects were more common in patients using systemic corticosteroids. They concluded that combined steroid injection and topical steroid treatment in IGM is as effective as systemic steroid treatment and this combination can be the first-line treatment approach with rare side effects.

In conclusion, intralesional steroid injection with concomitant topical steroid application can be used easily in patients with uncomplicated IGM, due to its ease of use and good patient compliance with satisfying results.

Methotrexate

In the treatment of IGM, methotrexate was first used in the 2000s [56, 83].

Kim et al. [83] initiated corticosteroid therapy as the first-line treatment in their patients with IGM. Although the initial response to corticosteroid therapy was good, the lesions recurred with the reduction of the corticosteroid dose. For the recurred lesions, the authors administered azathioprine first. Once the patient could not tolerate azathioprine, they started methotrexate at a dose of 10 mg/week and then increased the dosage to 15 mg/week which was continued for 12 months. They did not observe any serious side effects or recurrence in the patient. Based on their experience with the initial patient, the authors used methotrexate treatment with corticosteroids in three more patients. They reported that the duration of methotrexate use varied between 3 and 6 months, but two of three patients relapsed after 1–3 months of discontinuation of the drug. They concluded that methotrexate can be used for troublesome IGM patients to avoid corticosteroid-related side effects.

Katz et al. [56] used methotrexate (10 mg/week per oral, 12 months) due to the development of corticosteroid-induced diabetes mellitus in their first IGM patient. Methotrexate (7.5 mg per oral/week) was administered in another patient as a consequence of recurrence after the reduction of corticosteroid dose.

Until now, methotrexate has mostly been used for the treatment of patients with recurring or refractory IGM. This has been at different doses and durations [12, 13,

16, 52, 67, 70, 71, 84–87]. It has also been preferred as a maintenance therapy for IGM patients in remission with corticosteroids [88]. However, recently, there have been studies proposing methotrexate as a first-line therapy [13, 85, 87]. The commonly used dosage is 10–20 mg per oral/week.

In conclusion, methotrexate is effective in patients with IGM, and with once-a-week dosage, it is an easy-to-use drug. According to recent studies, methotrexate seems to be a treatment option in IGM, especially in patients with refractory or recurrent disease. However, patients should be monitored due to possible hematological side effects especially in the treatment of coexisting rheumatologic diseases.

Azathioprine

Azathioprine, a purine analogue and an immunosuppressive drug, is also used in some rheumatologic or autoimmune diseases such as rheumatoid arthritis, granulomatosis with polyangiitis, Crohn's disease, ulcerative colitis, and systemic lupus erythematosus. There is also little experience with azathioprine for the treatment of IGM [69, 87–89]. Azathioprine is usually used in combination with corticosteroids as a maintenance therapy to avoid the side effects of corticosteroids.

The most comprehensive study with the use of azathioprine for the treatment of IGM is by Konan et al. [89]. The authors administered azathioprine at a dose of 150 mg/day with corticosteroid in 14 IGM patients. They decreased both the corticosteroid and azathioprine doses over time and the treatment period lasted for 6–24 months. As a result, they concluded that the addition of azathioprine to corticosteroid allows reduction of corticosteroid doses and may increase the success of the treatment with lower steroid-related side effects.

Mycophenolate Mofetil

In an IGM patient refractory to corticosteroid and methotrexate therapy, mycophenolate mofetil, an immunosuppressive drug that inhibits inosine monophosphate dehydrogenase, and intralesional injections of triamcinolone acetonide were used. The study emphasized the effectiveness of mycophenolate mofetil in IGM treatment [90].

In summary, in order to conclude that mycophenolate mofetil is effective in IGM treatment, further research such as reporting the use of mycophenolate mofetil as a single agent are needed.

1.1.5 Traditional Treatment

In an interesting traditional medicine study by Xue et al. [91], the efficacy of "Chuang Ling Ye," a traditional Chinese herbal medicine compound, was investigated for the treatment of IGM. The authors found a statistically significant decrease in the mass size and pain scores in IGM patients who were administered Chuang

Ling Ye. Also, the expression of interleukin-1β, interferon-γ, and tumor necrosis factor-α levels reduced in these patients.

In another interesting traditional medicine study, IGM patients were divided into two groups: patients who underwent surgery only and those who underwent surgery plus "Yanghe decoction," a traditional Chinese herbal formulation which has various anti-inflammatory effects. Yanghe decoction was applied to the patients daily, 30 minutes after breakfast and after dinner for 3 months. It has been reported that patients who were administered Yanghe decoction achieved complete remission in a shorter time, had a higher rate of complete remission, and had lower recurrence rates [92].

Yuksekdag [76] published an article about the efficacy of St. John's-wort (*Hypericum perforatum*) oil for intractable skin lesions of patients with IGM. Oil massage was recommended after the complete regression of granulomatous mass with oral steroid therapy. Although the study group is small and the oil massage was not the only treatment modality, it seems to be effective which may be due to two important constituents of St. John's-wort oil, hypericin and hyperforin, which are proven to have antimicrobial, anti-inflammatory, and antioxidant effects.

A traditional and complementary medicine treatment recommendation has been revealed by Caliskan et al. [93] by using medicinal leeches and cupping therapy on 30 patients with IGM. They stated that symptoms had completely resolved within mean 110.3 days and complete radiologic response was confirmed 3 months after the end of the therapy. There was no relapse after the follow-up period of 22 months [93].

Recently, a case report from India was published with regards to the Ayurvedic management of IGM. This study reported that Ayurveda may be an effective treatment option with significantly fewer adverse effects compared with steroids and antibiotics and it may be used in both managements of symptoms and prevention of recurrence [94].

In conclusion, more evidence-based studies are required on traditional medicine practices for the treatment of IGM.

1.1.6 Others

Colchicine

Colchicine, a well-known drug for a long time, has been used in autoimmune and inflammatory diseases. Some mechanisms of action of colchicine are the inhibition of neutrophil activation and migration to inflammation sites, while inhibiting microtubule polymerization and thus inhibiting mitosis by binding to tubulins [95]. Although colchicine is used in IGM treatment generally in combination with other immunosuppressive drugs, there has been little evidence on dosing and effectivity [63, 69, 96–98].

Etanercept

In a patient with arthritis, erythema nodosum, and IGM, an NSAID was prescribed and no response was obtained in erythema nodosum and IGM; however, little improvement was seen in the arthritis findings. High-dose corticosteroid treatment was administered to the patient, but it was reported that only erythema nodosum healed in a short time, and there was no improvement in breast findings. There was also no improvement detected with the treatment of azathioprine and danazol. Thereafter, etanercept, a tumor necrosis factor inhibitor, was given at a dose of 50 mg every 2 weeks. Following this, the etanercept dose was tapered, and methotrexate was started. The patient, who remained in remission for 6 months, relapsed and etanercept was started again. In the light of these findings, the authors concluded that etanercept may be effective for the treatment of IGM [73].

Minocycline

The anti-inflammatory and immunomodulatory activities of minocycline, a tetracycline group antibiotic, have been demonstrated in different ways [99]. In the treatment of IGM, minocycline was included in only a case report [60].

Platelet-Rich Plasma

Platelet-rich plasma (PRP) is an autologous concentration of human platelets that contains many growth factors actively secreted by platelets as platelet-derived growth factor, transforming growth factor, vascular endothelial growth factor, and epithelial growth factor to initiate wound healing. It also contains cell adhesion molecules like fibronectin. The clinical application of PRP in sports, spine, and musculoskeletal medicine has soared in the last decade. Starting from its efficacy in these areas of medicine, we planned to use it for a patient with a refractory and recurrent IGM with multiple ulcers and fistulae. After cleaning the wound with saline, PRP was applied and dressings were checked daily and the procedure was repeated if needed. On the tenth day of treatment, an obvious recovery in the wound was achieved. It sounds to be a promising treatment option with no known side effects; however, a large number of series are required [100].

Conclusion

Despite these findings, IGM still remains a mystery. Until the etiopathogenesis is fully understood, it seems that the continuation of symptomatic treatment will be the first-line treatment. The only tool we have to guide this mysterious illness is classification schemes. The scheme below may help to classify the disease according to symptoms and suggest treatment strategies (Fig. 1).

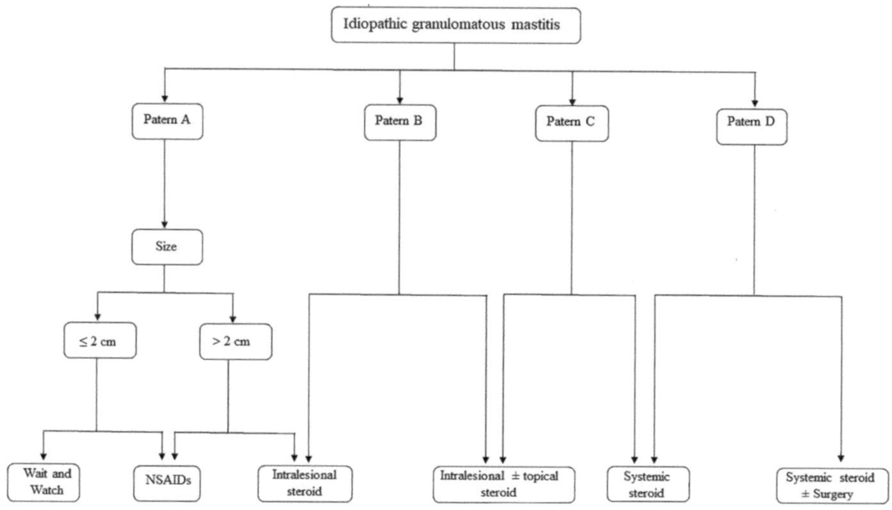

Fig. 1 An overview of treatment approaches in IGM

Treatment of IGM Patients with Erythema Nodosum

It is well known that patients with IGM may have extramammary manifestations such as erythema nodosum, arthralgia/arthritis, or episcleritis [17, 41, 101]. An ideal treatment approach has not yet been established in IGM patients with erythema nodosum, like in all IGM patients [41, 43, 45, 69, 85, 98, 102–107]. Most of the literature on this subject is in the form of case reports. Although it has been reported that different corticosteroids have been successfully used with different doses in these patients, there have been some patients who do not respond to treatment or have recurrence when the corticosteroid dose is tapered.

In the study by Akın et al. [41] which is one of the three important studies, they reported that they achieved complete response in all their patients with a relatively high dose of methylprednisolone treatment and no recurrence was observed. However, in a case report where the same drug was used at the same dose, it was reported that no response was obtained [105]. In another study comparing IGM patients with and without erythema nodosum, they reported success rates of 50% and 75%, respectively, and recurrence rates of 25% and 17.4%, respectively [45]. In the final important study on this subject, they emphasized that methotrexate treatment could be a useful option in IGM patients with systemic inflammation findings such as erythema nodosum and/or arthritis [85].

In conclusion, although there is little experience in the treatment of IGM patients with erythema nodosum, it is generally believed that corticosteroid therapy is successful. Methotrexate may be also useful in patients who do not achieve the desired success with steroids or in patients with recurrence. However, it is a fact that prospective studies are also needed.

Treatment of IGM Patients with Pregnancy

Idiopathic granulomatous mastitis is not common during pregnancy, but if it exists, it is usually diagnosed in the second or third trimester. Erythema nodosum and/or arthritis is also more common in these patients than in IGM patients who are not pregnant. The patients being pregnant at the time of diagnosis constitute 4.5% to 9% of all IGM patients [17, 24]. Literature in IGM treatment in pregnant women is very limited [48, 81, 89, 106, 108, 109]. Two approaches draw attention in pregnant IGM patients, one of them is observation, and the other is corticosteroids. Due to the possible side effects of the drugs on both the patient and the fetus, it is generally thought that medical treatment should be avoided or postponed. But antenatal corticosteroid administration is well known to prevent respiratory stress, especially at fetuses at risk of early-term labor. Therefore, systemic or local corticosteroids (intralesional administration or topical) can be an option in pregnant patients, especially in the third trimester within the knowledge of the patient's obstetrician against the risk of surrenal gland suppression in the fetus. However, this research area also requires further studies.

2 Prognosis

Idiopathic granulomatous mastitis is a benign inflammatory breast disease that is self-limited and can achieve self-remission [17, 23, 26]. Various studies have reported different recurrence rates in IGM patients, depending on the treatment approaches [11, 37, 110–112]. The overall recurrence rate independent of treatment ranges from 16.2% to 29.1% [37, 112].

In a highly comprehensive study by Kaviani et al. [37], according to treatment approaches, regarding the recurrence rates for observation, nonsteroidal anti-inflammatory drugs, corticosteroids, antibiotics, methotrexate, and surgery (open drainage, incision biopsy and open drainage, excision biopsy, and breast-conserving surgery) were 12.9%, 16.9%, 24.8%, 12.5%, 8.3%, and 48.7%, respectively.

In a meta-analysis by Godazandeh et al. [11], 559 IGM patients were included, and the overall recurrence rate was 13.2% for all patients, while this rate was 17.7% in patients who received corticosteroid therapy, 8.7% in patients who underwent surgery alone, and 3.2% in patients who had surgery and steroid therapy together.

Studies on factors affecting recurrence in IGM are limited. Azizi et al. [110] showed the only factor significantly associated with the recurrence was the presence of skin lesions on affected breasts. Çetinkaya et al. [113] found that the recurrence rate was high in patients with high neutrophil to lymphocyte ratio (>5.02). The most important limitation for this study is the low number of IGM patients, especially the ones with recurrence.

In the multicenter study by Uysal et al. [112], 750 IGM patients were reviewed. The percentages of the first recurrence and re-recurrence were 17% and 3%, respectively. They found statistical relationships between recurrence and pregnancy, breastfeeding, smoking, and history of breast infection in IGM patients.

Yilmaz et al. [75] used a scoring system that could be useful in predicting the recurrence of IGM. In this scoring system, parameters including number of births, duration of lactation, body mass index, luminal inflammation score, existence of fistula, and abscess/collection in ultrasonography were used. In this study the most important limitation is the small sample size of IGM patients with recurrence.

Idiopathic granulomatous mastitis is also a disease of secondary complications such as infection and delayed wound healing.

In conclusion, IGM is an inflammatory breast disease that can sometimes be controlled with a "wait-and-watch strategy" approach alone or sometimes with using different treatment options such as immunosuppressive drugs. For reasons unknown, this disease can remain dormant for a long period of time before recurrence. It is perhaps important to maintain long-term follow-up but no measure for prevention has been advised. However, recurrences are important complications, and more studies, especially prospective ones, are required describing appropriate and effective treatment strategies for patients with recurring IGM.

References

1. Altintoprak F, Kivilcim T, Ozkan OV. Aetiology of idiopathic granulomatous mastitis. World J Clin Cases. 2014;2:852–8. https://doi.org/10.12998/wjcc.v2.i12.852.
2. Baslaim MM, Khayat HA, Al-Amoudi SA. Idiopathic granulomatous mastitis: a heterogeneous disease with variable clinical presentation. World J Surg. 2007;31:1677–81. https://doi.org/10.1007/s00268-007-9116-1.
3. Benson JR, Dumitru D. Idiopathic granulomatous mastitis: presentation, investigation and management. Future Oncol. 2016;12:1381–94. https://doi.org/10.2217/fon-2015-0038.
4. Yin Y, Liu X, Meng Q, Han X, Zhang H, Lv Y. Idiopathic granulomatous mastitis: etiology, clinical manifestation, diagnosis and treatment. J Investig Surg. 2022;35:709–20. https://doi.org/10.1080/08941939.2021.1894516.
5. Gulluoglu BM. Idiopathic granulomatous mastitis: do we really regard it as a surgical disease anymore? World J Surg. 2015;39:2724–5. https://doi.org/10.1007/s00268-015-3185-3.
6. Koksal H, Vatansev H, Artac H, Kadoglou N. The clinical value of interleukins-8, −10, and −17 in idiopathic granulomatous mastitis. Clin Rheumatol. 2020;39:1671–7. https://doi.org/10.1007/s10067-020-04925-8.
7. Moris D, Damaskos C, Davakis S, et al. Is idiopathic granulomatous mastitis a surgical disease? The jury is still out. Ann Transl Med. 2017;5:309. https://doi.org/10.21037/atm.2017.05.24.
8. Saydam M, Yilmaz KB, Sahin M, Anik H, Akinci M, Yilmaz I, et al. New findings on autoimmune etiology of idiopathic granulomatous mastitis: serum IL-17, IL-22 and IL-23 levels of patients. J Investig Surg. 2020;34:993–7. https://doi.org/10.1080/08941939.2020.1725190.
9. Ucaryilmaz H, Koksal H, Emsen A, Kadoglou N, Dixon JM, Artac H. The role of regulatory T and B cells in the etiopathogenesis of idiopathic granulomatous mastitis. Immunol Investig. 2022;51:357–67. https://doi.org/10.1080/08820139.2020.1832114.

10. Cetin K, Sıkar HE, Goret NE, Rona G, Barışık NÖ, Küçük HF, et al. Comparison of topical, systemic, and combined therapy with steroids on idiopathic granulomatous mastitis: a prospective randomized study. World J Surg. 2019;43:2865–73. https://doi.org/10.1007/s00268-019-05084-x.

11. Godazandeh G, Shojaee L, Alizadeh-Navaei R, Hessami A. Corticosteroids in idiopathic granulomatous mastitis: a systematic review and meta-analysis. Surg Today. 2021; https://doi.org/10.1007/s00595-021-02234-4.

12. Haddad M, Sheybani F, Arian M, Gharib M. Methotrexate-based regimen as initial treatment of patients with idiopathic granulomatous mastitis. Breast J. 2020;26:325–7. https://doi.org/10.1111/tbj.13590.

13. Kehribar DY, Duran TI, Polat AK, Ozgen M. Effectiveness of methotrexate in idiopathic granulomatous mastitis treatment. Am J Med Sci. 2020;360:560–5. https://doi.org/10.1016/j.amjms.2020.05.029.

14. Mansy AM, Abdellatif A, Abdel-Hadi M, Abou Elnagah G, El Messiry M. Study of clinico-pathological changes before and after corticosteroid therapy in cases of idiopathic granulomatous mastitis. Breast J. 2021;27:486–8. https://doi.org/10.1111/tbj.14215.

15. Montazer M, Dadashzadeh M, Moosavi Toomatari SE. Comparison of the outcome of low dose and high-dose corticosteroid in the treatment of idiopathic granulomatous mastitis. Asian Pac J Cancer Prev. 2020;21:993–6. https://doi.org/10.31557/APJCP.2020.21.4.993.

16. Postolova A, Troxell ML, Wapnir IL, Genovese MC. Methotrexate in the treatment of idiopathic granulomatous mastitis. J Rheumatol. 2020;47:924–7. https://doi.org/10.3899/jrheum.181205.

17. Koksal H. What are the new findings with regard to the mysterious disease idiopathic granulomatous mastitis? Surg Today. 2021;51:1158–68. https://doi.org/10.1007/s00595-020-02204-2.

18. Wolfrum A, Kummel S, Theuerkauf I, Pelz E, Reinisch M. Granulomatous mastitis: a therapeutic and diagnostic challenge. Breast Care (Basel). 2018;13:413–8. https://doi.org/10.1159/000495146.

19. Irkorucu O. Granulomatous mastitis: a practical classification system. Isr Med Assoc J. 2016;18:307–8.

20. Irkorucu O. Granulomatous mastitis: we need a useful classification system. Am J Surg. 2018;216:642. https://doi.org/10.1016/j.amjsurg.2017.08.007.

21. Yaghan R, Hamouri S, Ayoub NM, Yaghan L, Mazahreh T. A proposal of a clinically based classification for idiopathic granulomatous mastitis. Asian Pac J Cancer Prev. 2019;20:929–34. https://doi.org/10.31557/APJCP.2019.20.3.929.

22. Kaviani A, Vasigh M. Classification of the clinical presentation, severity, and response to treatment in idiopathic granulomatousis mastitis. Arch Breast Cancer [Internet]. 2021;8:1–3. https://doi.org/10.32768/abc.2021811-3.

23. Bouton ME, Jayaram L, O'Neill PJ, Hsu CH, Komenaka IK. Management of idiopathic granulomatous mastitis with observation. Am J Surg. 2015;210:258–62. https://doi.org/10.1016/j.amjsurg.2014.08.044.

24. Davis J, Cocco D, Matz S, Hsu CH, Brown MJ, Lee J, et al. Re-evaluating if observation continues to be the best management of idiopathic granulomatous mastitis. Surgery. 2019;166:1176–80. https://doi.org/10.1016/j.surg.2019.06.030.

25. Lai EC, Chan WC, Ma TK, Tang AP, Poon CS, Leong HT. The role of conservative treatment in idiopathic granulomatous mastitis. Breast J. 2005;11:454–6. https://doi.org/10.1111/j.1075-122X.2005.00127.x.

26. Cetinkaya OA, Celik SU, Terzioglu SG, Eroglu A. The predictive value of the neutrophil-to-lymphocyte and platelet-to-lymphocyte ratio in patients with recurrent idiopathic granulomatous mastitis. Eur J Breast Health. 2020;16:61–5. https://doi.org/10.5152/ejbh.2019.5187.

27. Korkut E, Akcay MN, Karadeniz E, Subasi ID, Gursan N. Granulomatous mastitis: a ten-year experience at a university hospital. Eurasian J Med. 2015;47:165–73. https://doi.org/10.5152/eurasianjmed.2015.118.

28. Kıvılcım T, Altıntoprak F, Memiş B, Ferhatoğlu MF, Kartal A, Dikicier E, et al. Role of bacteriological agents in idiopathic granulomatous mastitis: real or not? Eur J Breast Health. 2018;15:32–6. https://doi.org/10.5152/ejbh.2018.4249.

29. Aghajanzadeh M, Hassanzadeh R, Alizadeh Sefat S, Alavi A, Hemmati H, Esmaeili Delshad MS, et al. Granulomatous mastitis: presentations, diagnosis, treatment and outcome in 206 patients from the north of Iran. Breast. 2015;24:456–60. https://doi.org/10.1016/j.breast.2015.04.003.

30. Li J. Diagnosis and treatment of 75 patients with idiopathic lobular granulomatous mastitis. J Investig Surg. 2019;32:414–20. https://doi.org/10.1080/08941939.2018.1424270.

31. Farouk O, Abdelkhalek M, Abdallah A, Shata A, Senbel A, Attia E, et al. Rifampicin for idiopathic granulomatous lobular mastitis: a promising alternative for treatment. World J Surg. 2017;41:1313–21. https://doi.org/10.1007/s00268-016-3857-7.

32. Salehi M, Salehi H, Moafi M, Aleban R, Tabatabaei SA, Salehi M, et al. Comparison of the effect of surgical and medical therapy for the treatment of idiopathic granulomatous mastitis. J Res Med Sci. 2014;19(Suppl 1):S5-8.

33. Salehi M, Salehi M, Kalbasi N, Hakamifard A, Salehi H, Salehi MM, et al. Corticosteroid and azithromycin in idiopathic granulomatous mastitis. Adv Biomed Res. 2017;6:8. https://doi.org/10.4103/2277-9175.199259.

34. Boufettal H, Essodegui F, Noun M, Hermas S, Samouh N. Idiopathic granulomatous mastitis: a report of twenty cases. Diagn Interv Imaging. 2012;93:586–96. https://doi.org/10.1016/j.diii.2012.04.028.

35. Hmissa S, Sahraoui W, Missaoui N, et al. Lobular idiopathic granulomatous mastitis. About 10 cases. Tunis Med. 2006;84:353–7.

36. Kaviani A, Noveiry BB, Jamei K, Rabbani A. How to manage idiopathic granulomatous mastitis: suggestion of an algorithm. Breast J. 2014;20:110–2. https://doi.org/10.1111/tbj.12216.

37. Kaviani A, Vasigh M, Omranipour R, Mahmoudzadeh H, Elahi A, Farivar L, et al. Idiopathic granulomatous mastitis: looking for the most effective therapy with the least side effects according to the severity of the disease in 374 patients in Iran. Breast J. 2019;25:672–7. https://doi.org/10.1111/tbj.13300.

38. Mizrakli T, Velidedeoglu M, Yemisen M, Mete B, Kilic F, Yilmaz H, et al. Corticosteroid treatment in the management of idiopathic granulomatous mastitis to avoid unnecessary surgery. Surg Today. 2015;45:457–65. https://doi.org/10.1007/s00595-014-0966-5.

39. DeHertogh DA, Rossof AH, Harris AA, Economou SG. Prednisone management of granulomatous mastitis. N Engl J Med. 1980;303:799–800. https://doi.org/10.1056/NEJM198010023031406.

40. Akcan A, Oz AB, Dogan S, Akgün H, Akyüz M, Ok E, et al. Idiopathic granulomatous mastitis: comparison of wide local excision with or without corticosteroid therapy. Breast Care (Basel). 2014;9:111–5. https://doi.org/10.1159/000360926.

41. Akın M, Karabacak H, Esendağlı G, Yavuz A, Gültekin S, Dikmen K, et al. Coexistence of idiopathic granulomatous mastitis and erythemanodosum: successful treatment with corticosteroids. Turk J Med Sci. 2017;47:1590–2. https://doi.org/10.3906/sag-1611-100.

42. Atak T, Sagiroglu J, Eren T, Ali Ozemir I, Alimoglu O. Strategies to treat idiopathic granulomatous mastitis: retrospective analysis of 40 patients. Breast Dis. 2015;35:19–24. https://doi.org/10.3233/BD-140373.

43. Binesh F, Shiryazdi M, Bagher Owlia M, Azimi S. Idiopathic granulomatous mastitis, erythema nodosum and bilateral ankle arthritis in an Iranian woman. BMJ Case Rep. 2013;2013:bcr2012007636. https://doi.org/10.1136/bcr-2012-007636.

44. Casteren CV, Jacquemyn Y, Himpe E, Verslegers I. Idiopathic ganulomatous mastitis. BMJ Case Rep. 2012;2012:bcr2012006187. https://doi.org/10.1136/bcr-2012-006187.

45. Cetin K, Sikar HE, Gulluoglu BM. Idiopathic granulomatous mastitis with erythema nodosum: is it a variant of clinical presentation indicating treatment resistance? A retrospective cohort study. Breast J. 2020;26:1645–51. https://doi.org/10.1111/tbj.13944.

46. Chirappapha P, Thaweepworadej P, Supsamutchai C, Biadul N, Lertsithichai P. Idiopathic granulomatous mastitis: a retrospective cohort study between 44 patients with different treatment modalities. Ann Med Surg (Lond). 2018;36:162–7. https://doi.org/10.1016/j.amsu.2018.11.001.

47. Deng JQ, Yu L, Yang Y, et al. Steroids administered after vacuum-assisted biopsy in the management of idiopathic granulomatous mastitis. J Clin Pathol. 2017;70:827–31. https://doi.org/10.1136/jclinpath-2016-204287.

48. Erozgen F, Ersoy YE, Akaydin M, Memmi N, Celik AS, Celebi F, et al. Corticosteroid treatment and timing of surgery in idiopathic granulomatous mastitis confusing with breast carcinoma. Breast Cancer Res Treat. 2010;123:447–52. https://doi.org/10.1007/s10549-010-1041-6.

49. Gopalakrishnan Nair C, Hiran JP, Menon RR, Misha. Inflammatory diseases of the non-lactating female breasts. Int J Surg. 2015;13:8–11. https://doi.org/10.1016/j.ijsu.2014.11.022.

50. Goulabchand R, Perrochia H, Aubert-Bringer E, Do Trinh P, Guilpain P. Idiopathic granulomatous mastitis responding to oral prednisone. Breast J. 2020;26:281–3. https://doi.org/10.1111/tbj.13552.

51. Gudimani SC, Rohit KC, Mithun VV, Gowda CK, Deepa AB. Idiopathic granulomatous mastitis: diagnostic and therapeutic challenges to general surgeon. Breast Dis. 2015;35:67–72. https://doi.org/10.3233/BD-140375.

52. Hashmi D, Al Samaraee A, Marks B, Fasih T. Idiopathic granulomatous mastitis: a diagnostic dilemma. Br J Hosp Med (Lond). 2020;81:1–4. https://doi.org/10.12968/hmed.2019.0287.

53. Hugon-Rodin J, Plu-Bureau G, Hugol D, Gompel A. Management of granulomatous mastitis: a series of 14 patients. Gynecol Endocrinol. 2012;28:921–4. https://doi.org/10.3109/0951359 0.2012.683075.

54. Hwang MJ, Rogers A, Vidya R. Idiopathic granulomatous mastitis: rare but important. BMJ Case Rep. 2010;2010:bcr1020092334. https://doi.org/10.1136/bcr.10.2009.2334.

55. Karanlik H, Ozgur I, Simsek S, Fathalizadeh A, Tukenmez M, Sahin D, et al. Can steroids plus surgery become a first-line treatment of idiopathic granulomatous mastitis? Breast Care (Basel). 2014;9:338–42. https://doi.org/10.1159/000366437.

56. Katz U, Molad Y, Ablin J, Ben-David D, Paran D, Gutman M, et al. Chronic idiopathic granulomatous mastitis. Ann N Y Acad Sci. 2007;1108:603–8. https://doi.org/10.1196/annals.1422.063.

57. Lei X, Chen K, Zhu L, Song E, Su F, Li S. Treatments for idiopathic granulomatous mastitis: systematic review and meta-analysis. Breastfeed Med. 2017;12:415–21. https://doi.org/10.1089/bfm.2017.0030.

58. Lucas R, Gussman D, Polis RL, Rattigan MI, Matulewicz TJ. Idiopathic granulomatous mastitis with erythema nodosum simulating breast abscess in pregnancy: a case report. Obstet Med. 2014;7:37–9. https://doi.org/10.1177/1753495X13502474.

59. Mahmodlou R, Dadkhah N, Abbasi F, Nasiri J, Valizadeh R. Idiopathic granulomatous mastitis: dilemmas in diagnosis and treatment. Electron Physician. 2017;9:5375–9. https://doi.org/10.19082/5375.

60. Mathew M, Siwawa P, Misra S. Idiopathic granulomatous mastitis: an inflammatory breast condition with review of the literature. BMJ Case Rep. 2015;2015:bcr2014208086. https://doi.org/10.1136/bcr-2014-208086.

61. Mathew Thomas V, Alexander SA, Bindal P, Vredenburgh J. Idiopathic granulomatous mastitis-a mystery yet to be unraveled: a case series and review of literature. Cureus. 2020;12:e6895. https://doi.org/10.7759/cureus.6895.

62. Naraynsingh V, Hariharan S, Dan D, Harnarayan P, Teelucksingh S. Conservative management for idiopathic granulomatous mastitis mimicking carcinoma: case reports and literature review. Breast Dis. 2010;31:57–60. https://doi.org/10.3233/BD-2009-0294.

63. Néel A, Hello M, Cottereau A, et al. Long-term outcome in idiopathic granulomatous mastitis: a western multicentre study. QJM. 2013;106:433–41. https://doi.org/10.1093/qjmed/hct040.

64. Olsen ML, Dilaveri CA. Idiopathic granulomatous mastitis: a case report of breast abscess. BMJ Case Rep. 2011;2011:bcr0520114271. https://doi.org/10.1136/bcr.05.2011.4271.
65. Oran ES, Gurdal SO, Yankol Y, Öznur M, Calay Z, Tunacı M, et al. Management of idiopathic granulomatous mastitis diagnosed by core biopsy: a retrospective multicenter study. Breast J. 2013;19:411–8. https://doi.org/10.1111/tbj.12123.
66. Pandey TS, Mackinnon JC, Bressler L, Millar A, Marcus EE, Ganschow PS. Idiopathic granulomatous mastitis--a prospective study of 49 women and treatment outcomes with steroid therapy. Breast J. 2014;20:258–66. https://doi.org/10.1111/tbj.12263.
67. Ruiter AM, Vegting IL, Nanayakkara PW. Idiopathic granulomatous mastitis: a great imitator? BMJ Case Rep. 2010;2010:bcr0320102844. https://doi.org/10.1136/bcr.03.2010.2844.
68. Sakurai K, Fujisaki S, Enomoto K, Amano S, Sugitani M. Evaluation of follow-up strategies for corticosteroid therapy of idiopathic granulomatous mastitis. Surg Today. 2011;41:333–7. https://doi.org/10.1007/s00595-009-4292-2.
69. Salesi M, Karimifar M, Salimi F, Mahzouni P. A case of granulomatous mastitis with erythema nodosum and arthritis. Rheumatol Int. 2011;31:1093–5. https://doi.org/10.1007/s00296-009-1273-0.
70. Sheybani F, Sarvghad M, Naderi H, Gharib M. Treatment for and clinical characteristics of granulomatous mastitis. Obstet Gynecol. 2015;125:801–7. https://doi.org/10.1097/AOG.0000000000000734.
71. Skandarajah A, Marley L. Idiopathic granulomatous mastitis: a medical or surgical disease of the breast? ANZ J Surg. 2015;85:979–82. https://doi.org/10.1111/ans.12929.
72. Su FH, Liu SC, Suen JH, Chen DS, Lou SMA. Idiopathic granulomatous mastitis: a case successfully treated with a minimum dose of a steroid. Chang Gung Med J. 2005;28:431–5.
73. Wang ST, Lin JC, Li CF, Lee YH. A successful case of etanercept used for idiopathic granulomatous mastitis. Breast J. 2019;25:343–5. https://doi.org/10.1111/tbj.13219.
74. Yabanoglu H, Colakoglu T, Belli S, Aytac HO, Bolat FA, Pourbagher A, et al. A comparative study of conservative versus surgical treatment protocols for 77 patients with idiopathic granulomatous mastitis. Breast J. 2015;21:363–9. https://doi.org/10.1111/tbj.12415.
75. Yilmaz TU, Gurel B, Guler SA, Baran MA, Erşan B, Duman S, et al. Scoring idiopathic granulomatous mastitis: an effective system for predicting recurrence? Eur J Breast Health. 2018;14:112–6. https://doi.org/10.5152/ejbh.2018.3709.
76. Yuksekdag S. The efficacy of St. John's wort (SJW, hypericum perforatum) oil macerates on intractable skin lesions of patients with idiopathic granulomatous mastitis: preliminary results. Authorea. 2020; https://doi.org/10.22541/au.159110380.08798337.
77. Altintoprak F. Topical steroids to treat granulomatous mastitis: a case report. Korean J Intern Med. 2011;26:356–9. https://doi.org/10.3904/kjim.2011.26.3.356.
78. Gunduz Y, Altintoprak F, Tatli Ayhan L, Kivilcim T, Celebi F. Effect of topical steroid treatment on idiopathic granulomatous mastitis: clinical and radiologic evaluation. Breast J. 2014;20:586–91. https://doi.org/10.1111/tbj.12335.
79. Altintoprak F, Kivilcim T, Yalkin O, Uzunoglu Y, Kahyaoglu Z, Dilek ON. Topical steroids are effective in the treatment of idiopathic granulomatous mastitis. World J Surg. 2015;39:2718–23. https://doi.org/10.1007/s00268-015-3147-9.
80. Alper F, Karadeniz E, Guven F, Yilmaz Cankaya B, Ozden K, Akcay MN. The evaluation of the efficacy of local steroid administration in idiopathic granulomatous mastitis: the preliminary results. Breast J. 2020;26:309–11. https://doi.org/10.1111/tbj.13588.
81. Kornfeld HW, Mitchell KB. Management of idiopathic granulomatous mastitis in lactation: case report and review of the literature. Int Breastfeed J. 2021;16:23. https://doi.org/10.1186/s13006-021-00370-8.
82. Toktas O, Konca C, Trabulus DC, Soyder A, Koksal H, Karanlik H, et al. A novel first-line treatment alternative for noncomplicated idiopathic granulomatous mastitis: combined intralesional steroid injection with topical steroid administration. Breast Care (Basel). 2021;16:181–7. https://doi.org/10.1159/000507951.

83. Kim J, Tymms KE, Buckingham JM. Methotrexate in the management of granulomatous mastitis. ANZ J Surg. 2003;73:247–9. https://doi.org/10.1046/j.1445-1433.2002.02564.x.

84. Freeman CM, Xia BT, Wilson GC, Lewis JD, Khan S, Lee SJ, et al. Idiopathic granulomatous mastitis: a diagnostic and therapeutic challenge. Am J Surg. 2017;214:701–6. https://doi.org/10.1016/j.amjsurg.2017.07.002.

85. Ringsted S, Friedman M. A rheumatologic approach to granulomatous mastitis: a case series and review of the literature. Int J Rheum Dis. 2021;24:526–32. https://doi.org/10.1111/1756-185X.14065.

86. Schmajuk G, Genovese MC. First report of idiopathic granulomatous mastitis treated with methotrexate monotherapy. J Rheumatol. 2009;36:1559–60. https://doi.org/10.3899/jrheum.090091.

87. Tekgöz E, Çolak S, Çinar M, Yilmaz S. Treatment of idiopathic granulomatous mastitis and factors related with disease recurrence. Turk J Med Sci. 2020;50:1380–6. https://doi.org/10.3906/sag-2003-93.

88. Peña-Santos G, Ruiz-Moreno JL. Idiopathic granulomatous mastitis treated with steroids and methotrexate. Ginecol Obstet Mex. 2011;79:373–6.

89. Konan A, Kalyoncu U, Dogan I, Kiliç YA, Karakoç D, Akdogan A, et al. Combined long-term steroid and immunosuppressive treatment regimen in granulomatous mastitis. Breast Care (Basel). 2012;7:297–301. https://doi.org/10.1159/000341388.

90. Di Xia F, Ly A, Smith GP. Mycophenolate mofetil as a successful therapy for idiopathic granulomatous mastitis. Dermatol Online J. 2017;23:13030/qt51g1k0zm.

91. Xue JX, Ye B, Liu S, Cao SH, Bian WH, Yao C. Treatment efficacy of Chuang Ling Ye, a traditional Chinese herbal medicine compound, on idiopathic granulomatous mastitis: a randomized controlled trial. Evid Based Complement Alternat Med. 2020;2020:6964801. https://doi.org/10.1155/2020/6964801.

92. Zhang X, Li J, Hu XJ. Postoperative Yanghe decoction regimen improves outcomes for idiopathic granulomatous mastitis: a retrospective cohort study. Medicine (Baltimore). 2020;99:e23136. https://doi.org/10.1097/MD.0000000000023136.

93. Caliskan M, Altay A, Eren A, Atayoglu AT. An integrative approach for idiopathic granulomatous mastitis. Indian J Surg. 2020;83(suply 2):388–94. https://doi.org/10.1007/s12262-020-02170-6.

94. Balakrishnan M, Shibila K. Post-operative ayurvedic management of non-healing idiopathic granulomatous mastitis - a case report. J Ayurveda Integr Med. 2021;12:710–4. https://doi.org/10.1016/j.jaim.2021.06.023.

95. Dalbeth N, Lauterio TJ, Wolfe HR. Mechanism of action of colchicine in the treatment of gout. Clin Ther. 2014;36:1465–79. https://doi.org/10.1016/j.clinthera.2014.07.017.

96. Ayeva-Derman M, Perrotin F, Lefrancq T, Roy F, Lansac J, Body G. Idiopathic granulomatous mastitis. Review of the literature illustrated by 4 cases. J Gynecol Obstet Biol Reprod (Paris). 1999;28:800–7.

97. Vanovcanova L, Lehotska V, Machalekova K, Waczulikova I, Minarikova E, Rauova K, et al. Idiopathic granulomatous mastitis - a new approach in diagnostics and treatment. Neoplasma. 2019;66:661–8. https://doi.org/10.4149/neo_2019_190201N100.

98. Vural S, Ertop P, Ceyhan K, Şanli H. An unusual cause of oligoarthritis and erythema nodosum: idiopathic granulomatous mastitis. Arch Rheumatol. 2017;32:71–5. https://doi.org/10.5606/ArchRheumatol.2017.5952.

99. Park CS, Kim SH, Lee CK. Immunotherapy of autoimmune diseases with nonantibiotic properties of tetracyclines. Immune Netw. 2020;20:e47. https://doi.org/10.4110/in.2020.20.e47.

100. Koksal H, Atay A, Eren Karanis MI, Turan E, Dogru O. Is platelet rich plasma an alternative treatment in granulomatous mastitis? GMJ. 2017;28:142. https://doi.org/10.12996/gmj.2017.41.

101. Pouchot J, Damade R, Barge J, Gaudin H, Vinceneux P. Idiopathic granulomatous mastitis and extramammary manifestations. Arch Pathol Lab Med. 1995;119:680.

102. Alungal J, Abdulla MC, Narayan R. Idiopathic granulomatous mastitis with erythema nodosum and polyarthritis. Reumatismo. 2016;68:97–9. https://doi.org/10.4081/reumatismo.2016.844.
103. Fahmy J, Halabi-Tawil M, Bagot M, Tournant B, Petit A. Erythema nodosum during the course of idiopathic granulomatous mastitis. Ann Dermatol Venereol. 2015;142:46–9. https://doi.org/10.1016/j.annder.2014.09.009.
104. Gumus M, Akkurt ZM, Gumus H. Is erythema nodosum coexisting with lesions of the breast a suggestive sign for idiopathic granulomatous mastitis? Turk J Surg. 2018;34:71–3. https://doi.org/10.5152/turkjsurg.2017.3161.
105. Kalayci TO, Koruyucu MB, Apaydin M, Etit D, Varer M. Idiopathic granulomatous mastitis associated with erythema nodosum. Balkan Med J. 2016;33:228–31. https://doi.org/10.5152/balkanmedj.2015.150089.
106. Sener Bahce Z, Aktas H. Patients with idiopathic granulomatous mastitis accompanied by erythema nodosum. Int J Clin Pract. 2021;75:e13928. https://doi.org/10.1111/ijcp.13928.
107. Zabetian S, Friedman BJ, McHargue C. A case of idiopathic granulomatous mastitis associated with erythema nodosum, arthritis, and reactive cough. JAAD Case Rep. 2016;2:125–7. https://doi.org/10.1016/j.jdcr.2016.01.011.
108. Garcia-Rodiguez JA, Pattullo A. Idiopathic granulomatous mastitis: a mimicking disease in a pregnant woman: a case report. BMC Res Notes. 2013;6:95. https://doi.org/10.1186/1756-0500-6-95.
109. Li SB, Xiong Y, Han XR, Liu ZY, Lv XL, Ning P. Pregnancy associated granulomatous mastitis: clinical characteristics, management, and outcome. Breastfeed Med. 2021;16:759–64. https://doi.org/10.1089/bfm.2021.0023.
110. Azizi A, Prasath V, Canner J, Gharib M, Sadat Fattahi A, Naser Forghani M, et al. Idiopathic granulomatous mastitis: management and predictors of recurrence in 474 patients. Breast J. 2020;26:1358–62. https://doi.org/10.1111/tbj.13822.
111. Shojaee L, Rahmani N, Moradi S, Motamedi A, Godazandeh G. Idiopathic granulomatous mastitis: challenges of treatment in iranian women. BMC Surg. 2021;21:206. https://doi.org/10.1186/s12893-021-01210-6.
112. Uysal E, Soran A, Sezgin E, Granulomatous Mastitis Study Group. Factors related to recurrence of idiopathic granulomatous mastitis: what do we learn from a multicentre study? ANZ J Surg. 2018;88:635–9. https://doi.org/10.1111/ans.14115.
113. Çetinkaya G, Kozan R, Emral AC, Tezel E. Granulomatous mastitis, watch and wait is a good option. Ir J Med Sci. 2020;190:1117–22. https://doi.org/10.1007/s11845-020-02406-0.

Surgical Treatment

Hande Koksal

1 Surgical Procedures

In the treatment of IGM, surgical approaches are used more limitedly than in the past. However, surgery may still be considered especially in patients with large lesions (>5 cm), those who are unresponsive to corticosteroids and other immuno-suppressive drugs, or patients with frequent recurrences. Despite its rapid success, the disadvantages of surgical interventions are problematic wound healing, possible aesthetic complications, and unhindered risk of recurrence [1]. In recent years, with the increasing importance of autoimmunity and immune dysregulation in the etio-pathogenesis, the question of whether IGM is a surgical disease has started to be asked more frequently [2–8].

Generally, preferred surgical procedures are drainage (percutaneous drainage or open drainage), excision, breast-conserving surgery, and mastectomy [1, 9–12].

1.1 Drainage

Drainage is a common surgical intervention in IGM treatment, especially in patients with a collection or abscess [10, 13]. However, we can find the answer to the question "Should every patient with abscess-like appearance be drained?" in the study by Yuksekdag [14]. In their study, the authors applied antibiotic

H. Koksal (✉)
Department of General Surgery, Selcuk University, Faculty of Medicine, Konya, Türkiye

  153
H. Koksal, N. Kadoglou (eds.), *Idiopathic Granulomatous Mastitis*,
https://doi.org/10.1007/978-3-031-30391-3_12

treatment to smaller abscesses while performing drainage to abscesses ≥ 2 cm. While ultrasonography-guided percutaneous drainage is usually preferred, open drainage can also be used in some patients [10]. Whether drainage will be performed and, if so, whether percutaneous or open drainage choices should be evaluated on the basis of each patient. An empirical antibiotic therapy should also be prescribed for patients undergoing drainage in order to avoid secondary infections.

1.2 Excision

Excision with safe margins is also an important treatment option in IGM treatment. However, in recent years, especially the use of corticosteroids and other immuno-suppressive agents has become popular, and therefore, surgery is less preferred. The proportions of patients who undergo excision are quite variable [13, 15–18]. As mentioned earlier, excision is effective and the control of symptoms are rapid. However, problems related with wound healing and aesthetic concerns are important. In addition, recurrence may occur despite excision unfortunately and this tends to be more often than expected (even up to 25%) [19].

In conclusion, excision may be a treatment option in patients with IGM resistant to corticosteroid and other immunosuppressive therapy, those with frequent recurrences, or patients with just a small residual mass after all other symptoms have resolved.

1.3 Breast-Conserving Surgery

Breast-conserving surgery is another surgical approach in IGM treatment. However, more research on breast-conserving surgery in IGM patients is required as this area in the field is limited. Kaviani et al. [9] reported that this surgery was preferred in only 3.9% of IGM patients in their study. However, surgical methods are not specified in the paper.

When surgery is required, using the simplest oncoplastic surgery techniques especially volume displacement procedures, extended excisions can be performed and successful results can be achieved with favorable esthetic outcomes. Multiple simple surgical attempts can cause contour deformities; thus, complex oncoplastic surgical methods have become known in this manner (Fig. 1). Recurrence may remain as a safety concern but complete excisions by extended surgery is likely to minimize the risk of recurrence.

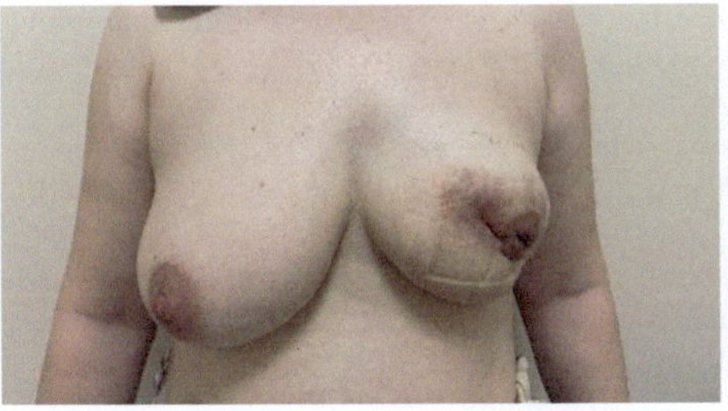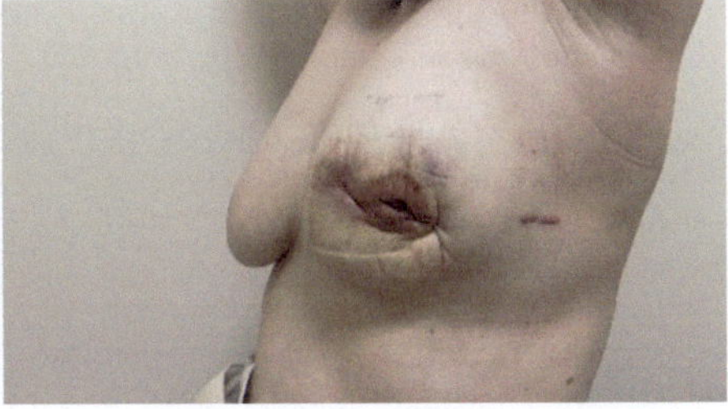

Fig. 1 A 47-year-old woman with IGM. Surgical resection of the inflamed tissue by simple extended excision resulted in contour deformity and nipple retraction

1.4 Mastectomy

The optimal path for treatment of this mysterious disease is still unclear. Long-lasting treatments with corticosteroids and antibiotics frequently reach the end with multiple wide local excisions in most patients. One of the most common problems in IGM patients is the high rate of recurrence. In patients who had undergone multiple surgical procedures with failure of conservative therapy modalities, radical treatment by mastectomy can be an option.

Apart from simple mastectomy, immediate reconstructions can also be performed by implant after skin-sparing mastectomy. Unfortunately, even as a case report, recurrences originated from residual breast tissue after subcutaneous mastectomy was reported and this underlined the necessity of radical mastectomy in certain patients [20]. Thus, radical approaches with mastectomy and primary flap reconstruction with autologous tissue was undertaken which offers a valuable option for safe, quick, and satisfactory aesthetic results with minimal recurrence rates. There is little evidence regarding the timing of reconstruction. Given the high rate of associated complications and recurrences, some authors believe that reconstruction should be undertaken as a delayed procedure to avoid potentially extensive surgery in the presence of inflammation and to allow completion of medical treatment [21].

Despite these surgical treatment options, IGM still remains a mystery. Until the etiopathogenesis is fully understood, it seems that the continuation of symptomatic and personalized treatment will be the first-line treatment.

References

1. Yin Y, Liu X, Meng Q, Han X, Zhang H, Lv Y. Idiopathic granulomatous mastitis: etiology, clinical manifestation, diagnosis and treatment. J Investig Surg. 2022;35:709–20. https://doi.org/10.1080/08941939.2021.1894516.

2. Ates D, Doner HC, Kurban S, Koksal H. The effect of soluble TREM-1 in idiopathic granulomatous mastitis. Immunol Investig. 2022;51:839–50. https://doi.org/10.1080/08820139.2021.1879846.

3. Emsen A, Koksal H, Ozdemir H, Kadoglou N, Artac H. The alteration of lymphocyte subsets in idiopathic granulomatous mastitis. Turk J Med Sci. 2021;51:1905–11. https://doi.org/10.3906/sag-2012-192.

4. Gulluoglu BM. Idiopathic granulomatous mastitis: do we really regard it as a surgical disease anymore? World J Surg. 2015;39:2724–5. https://doi.org/10.1007/s00268-015-3185-3.

5. Koksal H, Vatansev H, Artac H, Kadoglou N. The clinical value of interleukins-8, −10, and −17 in idiopathic granulomatous mastitis. Clin Rheumatol. 2020;39:1671–7. https://doi.org/10.1007/s10067-020-04925-8.

6. Moris D, Damaskos C, Davakis S, et al. Is idiopathic granulomatous mastitis a surgical disease? The jury is still out. Ann Transl Med. 2017;5:309. https://doi.org/10.21037/atm.2017.05.24.

7. Saydam M, Yilmaz KB, Sahin M, Anik H, Akinci M, Yilmaz I, et al. New findings on autoimmune etiology of idiopathic granulomatous mastitis: serum IL-17, IL-22 and IL-23 levels of patients. J Investig Surg. 2020;34:993–7. https://doi.org/10.1080/08941939.2020.1725190.

8. Ucaryilmaz H, Koksal H, Emsen A, Kadoglou N, Dixon JM, Artac H. The role of regulatory T and B cells in the etiopathogenesis of idiopathic granulomatous mastitis. Immunol Investig. 2022;51:357–67. https://doi.org/10.1080/08820139.2020.1832114.

9. Kaviani A, Vasigh M, Omranipour R, Mahmoudzadeh H, Elahi A, Farivar L, et al. Idiopathic granulomatous mastitis: looking for the most effective therapy with the least side effects according to the severity of the disease in 374 patients in Iran. Breast J. 2019;25:672–7. https://doi.org/10.1111/tbj.13300.

10. Kaviani A, Vasigh M. Classification of the clinical presentation, severity, and response to treatment in idiopathic granulomatousis mastitis. Arch Breast Cancer [Internet]. 2021;8:1–3. https://doi.org/10.32768/abc.2021811-3.

11. Poovamma CU, Pais VA, Dolas SC, Prema M, Khandelwal R, Nisheena R. Idiopathic granulomatous mastitis: a rare entity with a variable presentation. Breast Dis. 2014;34:101–4. https://doi.org/10.3233/BD-130358.

12. Yabanoglu H, Colakoglu T, Belli S, Aytac HO, Bolat FA, Pourbagher A, et al. A comparative study of conservative versus surgical treatment protocols for 77 patients with idiopathic granulomatous mastitis. Breast J. 2015;21:363–9. https://doi.org/10.1111/tbj.12415.

13. Koksal H. What are the new findings with regard to the mysterious disease idiopathic granulomatous mastitis? Surg Today. 2021;51:1158–68. https://doi.org/10.1007/s00595-020-02204-2.

14. Yuksekdag S. The efficacy of St. John's wort (SJW, hypericum perforatum) oil macerates on intractable skin lesions of patients with idiopathic granulomatous mastitis: preliminary results. Authorea. 2020; https://doi.org/10.22541/au.159110380.08798337.

15. Chirappapha P, Thaweepworadej P, Supsamutchai C, Biadul N, Lertsithichai P. Idiopathic granulomatous mastitis: a retrospective cohort study between 44 patients with different treatment modalities. Ann Med Surg (Lond). 2018;36:162–7. https://doi.org/10.1016/j.amsu.2018.11.001.

16. Prasad S, Jaiprakash P, Dave A, Pai D. Idiopathic granulomatous mastitis: an institutional experience. Turk J Surg. 2017;33:100–3. https://doi.org/10.5152/turkjsurg.2017.3439.

17. Shojaee L, Rahmani N, Moradi S, Motamedi A, Godazandeh G. Idiopathic granulomatous mastitis: challenges of treatment in iranian women. BMC Surg. 2021;21:206. https://doi.org/10.1186/s12893-021-01210-6.

18. Wang ST, Lin JC, Li CF, Lee YH. A successful case of etanercept used for idiopathic granulomatous mastitis. Breast J. 2019;25:343–5. https://doi.org/10.1111/tbj.13219.

19. Shin YD, Park SS, Song YJ, Son SM, Choi YJ. Is surgical excision necessary for the treatment of granulomatous lobular mastitis? BMC Womens Health. 2017;17:49. https://doi.org/10.1186/s12905-017-0412-0.

20. Hladik M, Scheller T, Ensat F, Wechselberger G. Idiopathic granulomatous mastitis: successful treatment by mastectomy and immediate breast reconstruction. J Plast Reconstr Aesthet Surg. 2011;64:1604–7. https://doi.org/10.1016/j.bjps.2011.07.011.
21. Taghizadeh R, Shelley OP, Chew BK, Weiler-Mithoff EM. Idiopathic granulomatous mastitis: surgery, treatment, and reconstruction. Breast J. 2007;13:509–13. https://doi.org/10.1111/j.1524-4741.2007.00474.x.

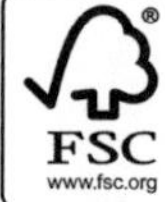

MIX
Papier aus verantwortungsvollen Quellen
Paper from responsible sources
FSC® C105338

If you have any concerns about our products,
you can contact us on
ProductSafety@springernature.com

In case Publisher is established outside the EU,
the EU authorized representative is:
**Springer Nature Customer Service Center GmbH
Europaplatz 3, 69115 Heidelberg, Germany**

Printed by Libri Plureos GmbH
in Hamburg, Germany